RISE & DEMISE OF THE CHIROPRACTIC PROFESSION

RISE & DEMISE OF THE CHIROPRACTIC PROFESSION

HOW ONE OF THE GREAT GIFTS
TO MANKIND WAS TAKEN TO ITS DEMISE
BY MIS-MANAGEMENT

R.B. Mawhiney, D.C., D.I.S.R.C.

Photos, newspaper excerpts and quotes, courtesy
of Volume I, 'History of Chiropractic in Wisconsin 1900-1950'
Volume II 'History of Chiropractic in Wisconsin 1950-1990.'

This book was printed in the United States of America.

To order additional copies of this book, contact:
Xlibris Corporation
1-888-795-4274
www.Xlibris.com
Orders@Xlibris.com
81324

CONTENTS

DEDICATION

I dedicate this book to all the young graduates

of chiropractic colleges so they may

realize if they do not understand the

history of their profession,

they will never know why

they are considered a second class

health care provider.

INTRODUCTION

One hundred thirteen years ago, a health care system was born as a profession by Daniel David Palmer of Davenport Iowa. Understanding the mentality of the people, the times, the education, social mores, economical positions, and a family environment, gives somewhat of an idea of how the people thought about their health. The Civil War had brought everyone's attention to the medical professions inability to treat day-to-day health problems. Sanitation, especially in the rural areas was not well understood.

A paid announcement carried in a New York paper in 1898 warned the population about the newest fad of immersing yourself in water for a period of time. This could spread diseases and infections, quoted the New York medical society as they warned all people to refrain from the practice. They were referring to the bathtub.

Two books that most families had in their home were the Bible and the medical book. The medical book had such information in the treatment of ailments as to inform the reader, if you suffer from consumption, dig a one square foot hole in the ground, place your face in the hole and breath. Another interesting one dealing with a systemic problem was to put hogs' fat on the bottom of your feet and hold them in front of the fireplace. The treatment for diabetes was to drink a lot of wine. People, familiar with home remedies, normally passed that information down through the family to treat most conditions. The importance of this new treatment procedure, chiropractic, was destined to be a Godsend to millions of people.

I entered into the profession a little over 50 years later, and as a young man listen to my professors and the older practitioners and learned about the early history of chiropractic. Even when I finished my internship, many states would not allow chiropractors to be called doctors and many states had no licensing laws for chiropractic. There was no insurance coverage and we as students were both surprised and concerned that our profession had not established itself more completely in the first half of the 20th-century. Most young professionals looked to the leaders of their profession, whether it is educational, geographical or national to provide the pathways for us to grow and to apply the knowledge that we had learned. I was not aware, upon graduation of how much dislike the average medical doctor had for Chiropractic and chiropractors in particular. World War II was over and the returning veterans were rushing to go to school.

The purpose of this book is to inform the reader why the chiropractic profession has not grown to its potential. In 113 years, there are approximately 55,000 practicing Chiropractors. There are approximately 550,000 medical doctors. Chiropractic remains the most beneficial, scientific, non-invasive, drugless healing art in the world. Over 100 years after its inception, there are many countries throughout the world that do not allow chiropractic practitioners. Something is wrong with this picture when millions of people have received benefits. Scientific articles have been published confirming the science of chiropractic and yet political leverage has prevented the profession from being available to the populace with its potential for relief of suffering.

The failure of the leaders in the profession to take advantage of all the opportunities available during the last century has regulated the profession to a second-class citizenship.

During the last 50 + years, I have been involved in testifying before state Senate's unctioning as an officer of state associations, involved in national organizations working within the academic structure and have seen the lack of assertiveness demonstrated over and over.

I am not as naive as to feel that the readers of this book will rise up, stimulate the leaders of the profession or to take on members of the establishment to bring about sweeping changes. I think the knowledge people acquire of why, one of the greatest boons to humanity's health and possible happiness, never made the grade.

Before his death, Bill Lucky, owner and publisher of Chiropractic Economics magazine, asked me to contribute an article in an 'opinion' column about my prediction for the chiropractic profession in the 21st century. I wrote that the chiropractic profession would be regulated to an ancillary health care provider, as are physical therapists. I gave my opinions as to why this would happen and he decided the article was too negative to be included in the publication.

I now give my opinion, as to why this all came about.

CHAPTER I

General History & Background

In the years following the Civil War, the population became very much aware of the problems in the medical field. The general opinion was that the medical doctor had three things in his little black bag. One was a meat saw; one was a cutting knife and opium or morphine. Soldiers wounded in the arms or legs knew they would be amputated since there was no treatment available.

Dr. Andrew Taylor Still was a frontier physician and became very concerned about the lack of treatment available for day-to-day ailments. Homeopathy was considered, since the 1700's, to be any procedure outside normal medical practice. Since medical practice may also include bleeding and drilling holes in the skull to relieve pressure headaches. Dr. Still was sure there was another way of treating health problems and founded what was to become the osteopathic profession. In general terms this meant utilizing heat, cold, electricity and general musculoskeletal manipulation. The philosophy, contrary to accepted medical practice, implied the body functions as a whole unit and was dependent upon circulation, nerve function and muscular activity in order to maintain health. The original practitioners of osteopathy did not utilize medications and they were classed as a drugless profession.

In 1895, Daniel David Palmer was classed as a 'magnetic healer'. He also fell into the category of homeopathy, being outside the medical field, which was not unusual at the time. Many individuals practiced various methods which were considered outside the normal medical field. D.D. Palmer, along with many others practicing some type of healing art, were offered an M.D. degree in the mid 1890's. He refused the degree continuing to practice magnetic healing. Tradition has stated that one day the janitor came into his room and having noted the man was deaf he volunteered to help him. the story is he noticed a lump in the man's neck and proceeded to apply pressure to the lump and surrounding area. Something moved in the man's neck and his hearing was restored.

As was common in those days, family treatment procedures, which may have been handed down through generations, were kept secret. He started investigating these particular responses and determined displacement of any of the vertebra could bring about dysfunction. In effect the chiropractic profession was born. Dr. Still's philosophy that malformations and malfunctions in the body systems were the cause of disease. D.D. Palmer surmised that God, not having made any mistakes, created the brain and nervous system first, which controlled the bodies function, would be the primary cause of malfunction. He began to refer to interference and the nervous system, through the spine, as dis-ease.

There were the allopathic physicians, homeopathic physicians and the alternative practitioners, at that time.

The populace was undoubtedly confused and obtained the services of anyone who could provide help.

D.D. Palmer's son, B.J. saw the possibility of extending this treatment procedure by spreading the word and starting a school as Dr. STILL had done. D.D. Palmer was not in favor of the idea but his son persisted.

Hippocrates, in ancient Greece, had said "look to the spine for disease". Though the medical profession takes the Hippocratic oath, they seem to have forgotten to look to the spine.

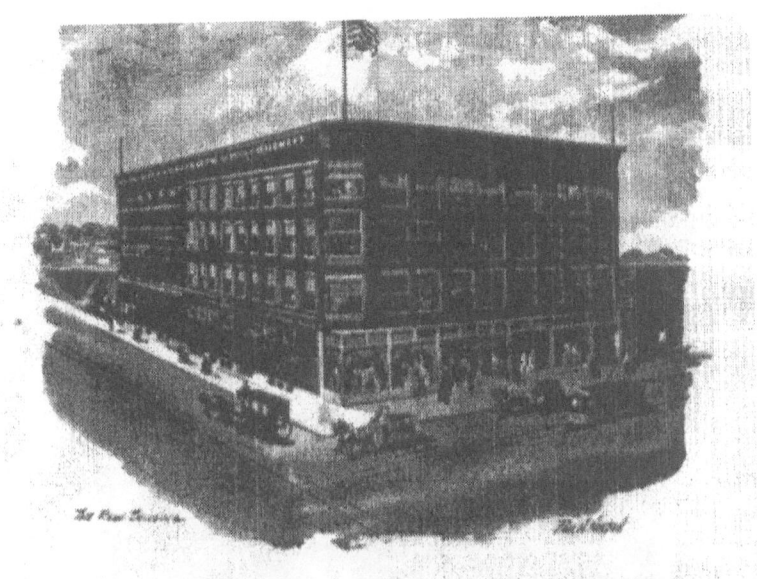

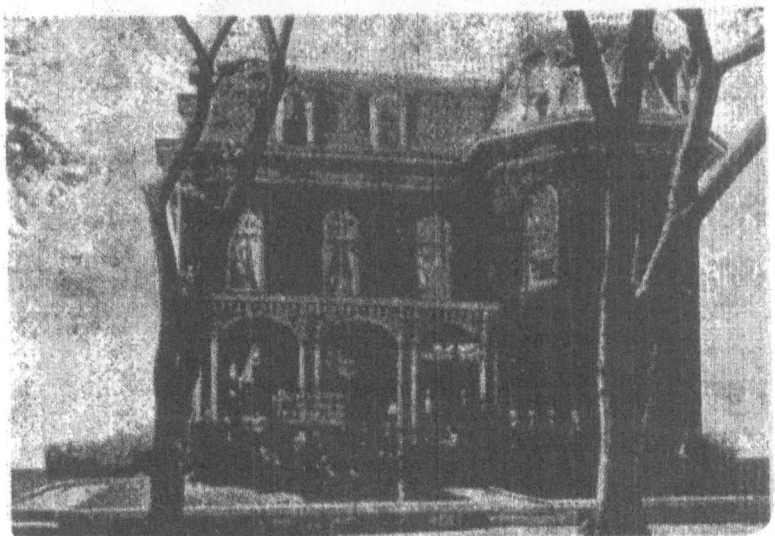

Top picture of D. D. Palmer office location
Bottom picture location of first school.

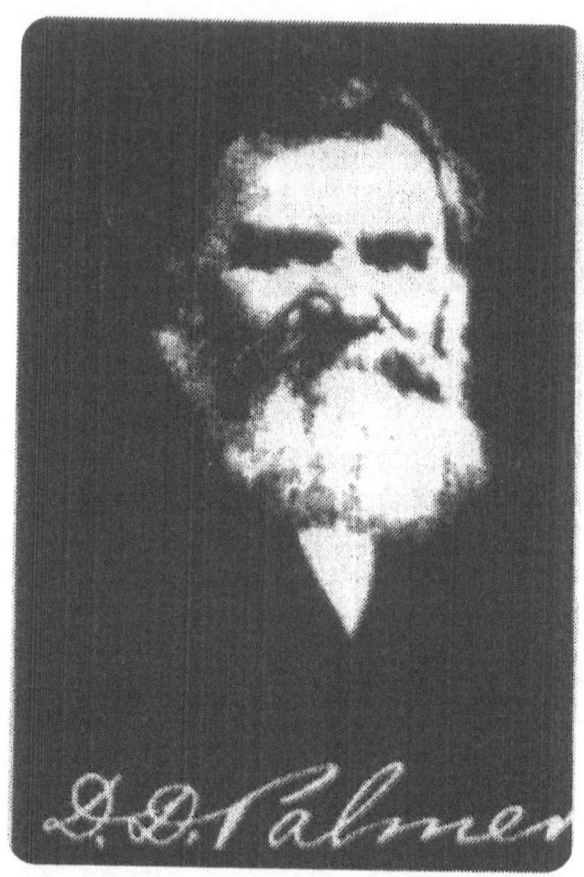

Dr. D. D. Palmer (Circa 1903)
"I have never found it to be beneath my dignity
to do anything to reduce human suffering"

In the beginning, D.D. Palmer did not want to share this information with anyone, but his son, B. J., convinced him that he should start a school. The first classes had six to nine individuals, many of them professionals such as teachers. The school is said to have started in 1899. An interesting aspect, as told by early graduates is that D. D. Palmer told those, who finished the course to "Go out and heal the suffering and teach".

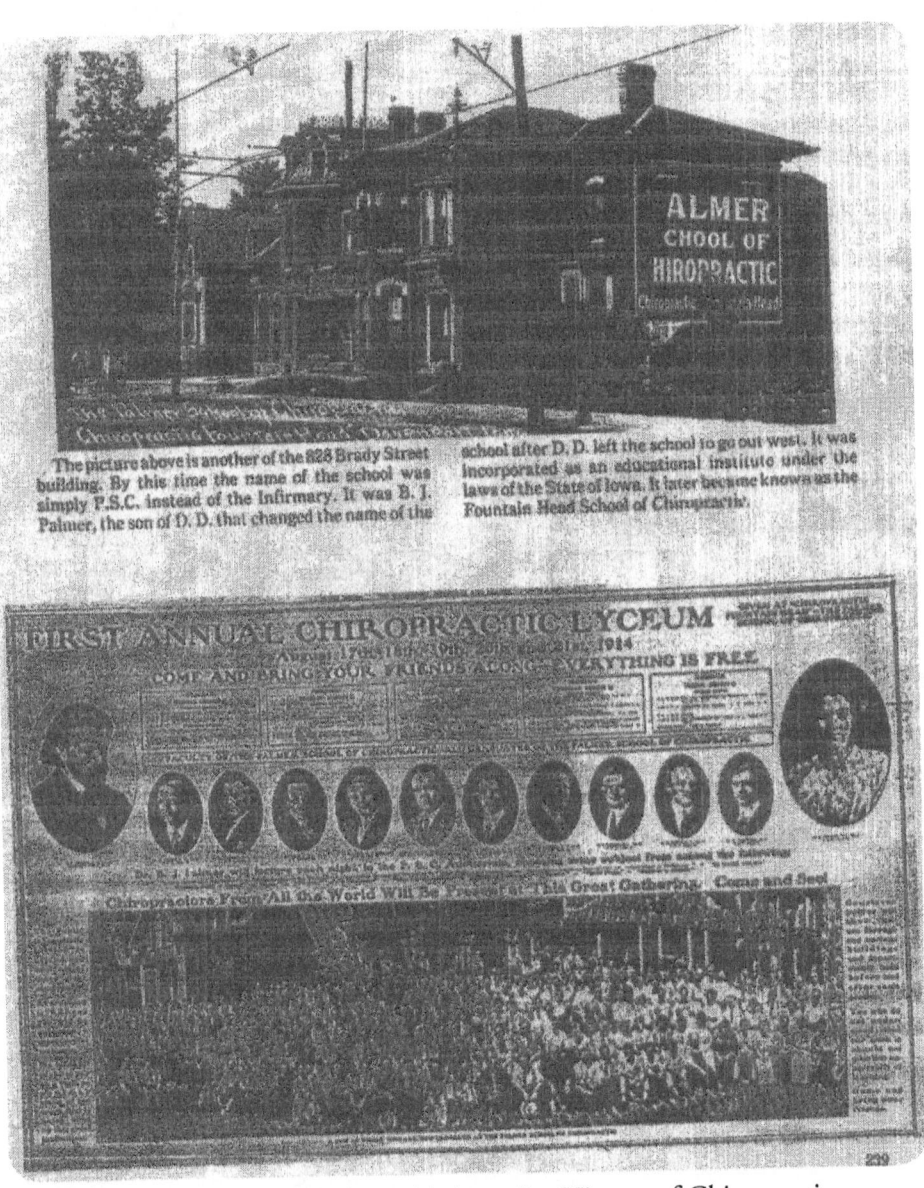

The picture above is another of the 828 Brady Street building. By this time the name of the school was simply P.S.C. instead of the Infirmary. It was B. J. Palmer, the son of D. D. that changed the name of the school after D. D. left the school to go out west. It was incorporated as an educational institute under the laws of the State of Iowa. It later became known as the Fountain Head School of Chiropractic.

Photo courtesy Roberts Publishing Co. History of Chiropractic
in Wisconsin 1900-1950 Vol. I

This would answer one of the question is as to why in 1906, when the school had the first lyceum, at the school, it has been told that 1000 chiropractor's attended. Therefore, what appeared to be happening was that Joe would teach uncle Henry and Sarah might teach cousin Sue, and each one would continue to teach as they practiced their new profession. There was no licensing, offices were in their homes and friends and relatives became the patients. The early problem was total lack of control or communication once they left the school. Anyone could put up a sign calling themselves the chiropractor even with less than six months of education. It's been reported that when D.D. Palmer was questioned by the Iowa state legislative body he told them he could teach anybody to be a chiropractor in 30 days. Politicians of the day were familiar with medical schools being attached to a state university and could not comprehend what he was saying. In D. D. Palmer's mind, displacement of the vertebra in the spine caused a malfunction of the nerve energy coming from the brain to innovate all the organs and tissues of the body. Since the word 'symptom' was from the Greek meaning sign, it meant any symptom was a sign something was wrong with the innervation causing the symptom to show up. He then conceived his opinion of being able to teach anyone to adjust the vertebra, in 30 days, and letting God's creation heal itself. When asked how the chiropractor would know what case to except he simply replied "If the patients are breathing, adjust them". He taught the students to look to the spine to find the nerve impingement, adjust the vertebra and allow the part the nerve enervated to bring about proper function.

Remember, that patients went to the doctor for conditions, which could not be treated at home. This new approach to treatment of their ailments opened up a new horizon. In a very short time, the medical profession became aware of the chiropractor's and determined to educate the population about the dangers of chiropractic.

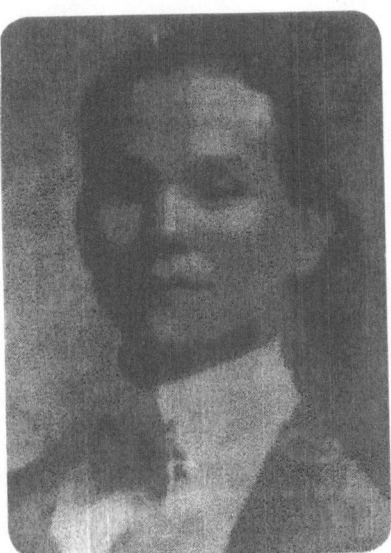

Dr. Shegataro Morikubo
1907

In 1907, a legal battle was taking place in La Cross Wisconsin involving a Japanese chiropractor. The year 1907 was a time when the U. S. was concerned with the possibility of war with Japan. Much was written in the newspapers across the country and a certain amount of interest was generated in the small town of La Cross Wisconsin. Dr. Morikubo was one of the earliest registered Chiropractors in the state and was called upon by the local newspaper to give some opinions as to his feelings about the possibility of war with Japan. According to the La Crosse Tribune, dated July 9, 1907 he was quoted as saying, "Japan will not go into a war with the United States unless it is necessary to protect its own country". Dr. Morikubo had his office in the Macmillan building and had been studying the conditions between the two countries ever since it started. Knowing the Japanese as he did and also the American public, after several years in this country, he believes that all talk about a war is a myth. It was not long after his second interview that some individuals in the community started to question his motives. The feeling was very anti Japanese and I do not know if it was the second installment in the July 10th 1907 issue of the Tribune, which triggered the next installment, but the Tribune headline on July 22nd 1907 read "Jap Chiropractor arrested today". Sub headline continued, "He was charged with practicing without a license. Jap will test state law". The medical doctor W. T. Sarles, chairman of the state medical board charged the chiropractor. The medical society further stated that the Japanese chiropractor was practicing as a chiropractor under an osteopathic license without identifying a difference between the two. Note: (The news report written by the reporter gave an insight into the thinking of the day)

"I am an American citizen duly naturalized and insist upon my American rights and liberty" said the little Jap with flashing eyes to this reporter.

The case went to trial as the "Wisconsin State Medical Society against Dr. Morikubo." There was a lot of news coverage, and in August, a jury, after 25 minutes of deliberation, came back with a not guilty verdict. Dr. W. T. Sarles indicated the medical profession would continue to persecute the chiropractor's until the Supreme Court could indicate that they could not be licensed. This was a warning sign to the profession of what was to happen in the future. The medical profession had issued a challenge indicating they would do whatever necessary to control the chiropractic profession. B.J. Palmer, the figurehead of the chiropractic profession did not recognize what was being done and the seeds were planted for the demise of the chiropractic profession.

Since the birth of chiropractic was in the Quad Cities area of Iowa, its growth continued in all directions of the compass from its center in Davenport. Individuals started coming to the Palmer school from Missouri, Minnesota, Wisconsin and Illinois. Unfortunately, the leaders of the profession, at that time were more concerned with developing their position and power than with the overall philosophy that D.D. Palmer had established.

Many early students were husbands and wives from small towns and many with only eighth grade educations. Though morally committed to the value of chiropractic, no plans were made for the development of the profession as a profession.

One of the basic problems was of course the lack of control over those who graduated from Palmer school. There was no licensing and there's no evidence that any effort was made to organize the profession on a state-to-state basis. The formation of the 30-60-90 club had been attributed to one of the Palmers. Since the medical profession had continued to harass the chiropractor's by having them arrested for practicing medicine without a license, they were being put in jail for 30-60 or 90 days. It became a badge of honor to be arrested and the club was formed for those who had the honor of being arrested. It was taken, by the leaders and the profession, as more of a joke then something that should be confronted. If it had not been for Dr. Morikubo of La Cross Wisconsin, giving the chiropractic profession a heads up as to what they could expect, no one could have traced the beginning of the demise of chiropractic.

Confusion concerning medical education, particularly in the rural areas made little concern to the population. Many medical practitioners were given a license to practice simply by serving as an apprentice to a physician. They may not have had any formal education beyond eighth grade.

CHAPTER II

Social Morays
Philosophy—Medical Image

During the first decade of the 20th century, there was a profusion of snake oil salesman, magnetic healers, osteopaths, chiropractor's, astrologers, palmists and individuals practicing crainiology. Therefore, the chiropractic profession was thrown into this mix of health-care providers. They moved along with the crowd. With no licensing involved and practicing in their homes, they felt immune to any type of regulation. The spirit of the phenomenal growth, of chiropractic, among the populace, actually contributed to the problems of the profession. If it would not have grown so quickly, it might have had more affect on the leaders in the college to help establish some type of professional control over what is practiced.

The medical profession had utilized the Hippocratic oath wherein they agreed to do no harm, continued to increase their image to the people by degrading other health care providers.

It is interesting to note how so many explanations and definitions change over the years. Over 60 years ago the general acceptance of the change from homeopathy to allopathic was considered quite clear. The homeopathic doctor tried to utilize natural herbs in the treatment of many ailments. At the turn-of-the-century the pharmaceutical companies began to exert more influence into the medical profession as the allopathic practitioner utilized pharmaceutical produced medications. Representatives of the pharmaceutical companies, detail men, started to introduce the medical profession to medications and the PDR (physicians desk reference), the

Bible by which medical doctors determined what medications to give the patient was introduced later.

The pharmaceutical companies began to improve the image of the medical profession and in so doing made them more cognizant of their sole ability to treat the sick. Following the arrest of Dr. Morikubo, the State Medical Societies began sending 'plants' into Chiropractic offices so they could arrest them for practicing medicine without a license. This procedure continued into the middle of the 20th-century. Those of us practicing in the 40's and '50's were still being arrested after being set up by these medical 'plants'. (Example) The person would make an appointment with the chiropractor and when asked what was wrong would make up some pain or discomfort. If the chiropractor accepted the patient's word and said for example "I will try to fix your headache", they could be arrested the next day for diagnosing, which falls into the realm of medical practice. I was fortunate because I received very good training in differential diagnosis. Those doctors who had only received 12 to 18 months of chiropractic education were not prepared to be aware that a patient might be making up the symptoms.

In many of the small towns in Minnesota, Iowa, Wisconsin, Illinois and Missouri, the chiropractor's dealing with 'hands on' procedure developed a very strong following. When the chiropractor was arrested in some of the smaller communities, it was not unusual for the local judge to have the chiropractor, if convicted of practicing medicine without a license, spend his time in jail on his day off and make arrangements for him to treat his patients in jail. Women chiropractors were not harassed or arrested to any degree. During my early years in practice, the local medical doctors expressed their dislike for the chiropractic profession in the local newspapers and particularly during the state medical convention. This harassment, by the 40's and 50's was well known by the colleges. Graduates were not informed of the reception they would receive when they opened a practice. A chiropractor could not be in the same building with a medical doctor. Neither a chiropractor nor osteopath could use any tax supported hospital facilities. They could not avail themselves of any medical research promoted by and funded by, the pharmaceutical companies.

Following the arrest of the Japanese doctor in La Cross Wisconsin, the medical profession increased the variety of attacks particularly by utilizing the media. During one of the state conventions, during the 1950's, the main speaker indicated he was able to buy a new car every year based on the number of chiropractic patients who came to him because of mistakes the chiropractor's had made. He indicated the chiropractor only had three months of education and consequently was a menace to the good people of the state. He said it was the responsibility of the medical doctor, who was the only one who knew how to treat the sick. It was their duty to protect the uninformed. He further stated that since the layman was totally ignorant of the aspects of disease and providing a cure, it was the total responsibility of the medical profession to protect those individuals. This tirades against the chiropractic profession was planted as front-page information in the local papers. Not once did any of the organizations, raise a finger or a voice in protest. It was noted that in the 60's and 70's as chiropractic was maturing clinically and academically, spokesmen for the profession did speak up in rebuttal to the statements. Unfortunately the Fountainhead of chiropractic, who did establish the standards by which the profession would operate, was B.J. Palmer, a true leader and promoter, who was apparently more concerned with the establishment of Palmer College as the epitome of chiropractic. With about 117 chiropractic schools by the early 1920's the situation had become unmanageable. The state's, through their legislative bodies, were not informed of the academic changes within the chiropractic profession. The increasing number of chiropractor's coming from the schools and a lack of any legislative control contributed to more confusion. It is the state legislators, in every state, who mandate the health care professions scope of practice.

In 1906, the National College of Chiropractic was started in Lombard Illinois. In 1911 the Wisconsin Chiropractic Association was begun. The numbers of chiropractors in Illinois or Wisconsin were few and with each state control by a legislative body, it was difficult to correlate the needs of the profession with each state.

The medical philosophy, by the early 1920's was based on the premise that disease was primarily a disruption of the chemical balance within the body and therefore would be treated by the addition of various chemical medications to balance the chemicals within the body. The chiropractic approach was based on the philosophy that God did not make any mistakes in putting the body together. Since the nervous system was the first system formed in embryo, all other structures were in direct relationship to the brain, spinal cord and the nervous system. Disruption of any transmission of the nerves, from the brain to a specific part, particularly where the nerve leaves the spine, is recognized. This will cause a malfunction of the part innervated bringing on disease. The chiropractor, by locating the area of the spine that housed the nerves, going to a specific part of the body, checked to determine if there was a vertebra out of position causing pressure on the nerve, decreasing normal nerve function to the part involved, and would adjust the vertebra into position.

When we look back 100 years, we can see how the medical, chiropractic and osteopathic professions were far less knowledgeable about the human body than they are today. The greatest advances in the medical profession have been in the areas of surgery involving organ transplants, brain surgery, microscopic surgery etc. The chiropractic profession in the last 100 years has increased its knowledge of the human body and its function but the specific treatment procedure remains the same. It was D.D. Palmer who coined the term 'Dis-ease'.

With the chiropractic profession, sending out graduate chiropractors with 6-12 and 18 months of education, the country did see a large influx of chiropractic practitioners across the United States. Because the philosophy was very easy to understand, based on the body's natural immunity and ability to renew itself, it was accepted by the population.

The medical profession, exposed to the same anatomical and neurological information dismissed it as quackery.

The flu epidemic of 1917 threw the United States into mass panic as the medical profession had no treatment procedures established. Many chiropractors had offices filled with patients with flu symptoms and early records, reported by doctors practicing at that time, recorded very few fatalities.

The same reaction was noted during the polio epidemic of the 1940's and 50's. The procedure followed by the medical profession when a patient was diagnosed with polio, was to observe them until paralysis was established and then provide rehabilitation therapy. I personally had an experience with a seven-year-old who was diagnosed as having polio. He was immediately subjected to chiropractic care and within five days was over the condition. When the parents told the medical doctor, he called it "spontaneous remission". The other term they used to circumvent chiropractic results was "misdiagnosis".

The profession was aware of these responses but was unable to receive any media coverage.

The medical profession, prior to the 1920's was able to inform the media that to protect them from charlton's they should have direct consultation with the local medical society, or a medical consultant, to screen any health advertisements or articles pertaining to treatment procedures. This way any article submitted to the media about chiropractic success in the treatment of conditions was stopped before it could be printed. This became standard procedure from the 1920's to this day.

State Organizations

By the 1930's and 40's, most states had established some type of state organization. Membership by the chiropractor's was not mandatory and therefore were not well attended. Since no pre chiropractic training, similar to Pre-med, had been established by the state legislature, most practicing chiropractors had little more than a high school diploma. The individuals running the state associations had little experience in operating the state organization. They did not recognize the battle that was necessary for them to bring to the population the benefits of chiropractic. They were not subsidized or aided in any way to promote research within the profession. Because of the harassment, they were more concerned in keeping themselves out of jail than compiling research data to present to the population.

The fault for this does lie with the early leaders in the profession. Graduates from medical schools, particularly in the Midwest, were encouraged to be members of the American Medical Association and state association, in order to qualify them for membership on the staff of a hospital. This control, since doctors needed the hospital, was an ideal method of control. I owned an office building in 1960 and was approached by a medical doctor wishing to rent space in the building. When an agreement was reached, she contacted the state medical society to give them her new address. They inquired as to other tenants, and when she told them there was a chiropractor in the building, she was informed she would not have hospital privileges if she rented at that location. The chiropractic profession recognized this control and did nothing to establish some type of control within the chiropractic profession. Granted there was little area available to provide such control but if the leaders would have established better legislative response to their dilemma, who knows what might have happened.

The schools in chiropractic were competitive. They were independently funded, primarily by tuition and public clinics. It was interesting to note that in the 1940's, if a resident in a midwest state wanted to be a veterinarian and there was no veterinarian college in their state, the state would provide their tuition for them to go to another state. If a resident wanted to go to a chiropractic college, there was no such tuition available. No effort was made by the state association to change this inequity.

Soon the profession initiated its next move towards second-class status. The medical image was constantly being enhanced, through the media, with unified promotions. The chiropractors, in turn, having formed state associations to help their image by getting better laws passed, decided to form separate state associations if they were unhappy with those in charge. The adage that has passed on through the years was 'if you don't like those running it, join, become active, and become an officer of the association and change things to your liking'. Some states had as many as four distinct state associations representing the profession. The leaders of these associations, were too ignorant to recognize that the state legislative bodies, who control their practice, would not take them serious as long as they could not agree among themselves. Whether this was a carryover from the mentality of the early century leaders advocating independence, or desire for personal control we will never know. The image of the profession was not taken seriously by the media, gatekeepers or legislators. When one group would make a stand on a political position, the other group would disagree.

When I had the privilege of testifying before a Senate committee and meeting in private with various legislators and governors, I had first' hand experience with their opinions as to the lack of leadership within the chiropractic profession. It was not until some states combined their many groups into one state association that proper legislative bills were passed.

One of the media releases that damaged the chiropractic profession was a news release "Patient dies from a broken neck after seeing a chiropractor for treatment". Patients who told their family medical doctor that they wanted see a chiropractor, they were reminded immediately of the patients who had suffered broken necks.

Once again, no massive rebuttal was put forth by the state associations. Over 100 years later, you will still hear some medical practitioners quoting that report which was never substantiated.

During the 1930's, 40's, and 50's, local medical societies decided to send in more medical plants so that more chiropractor's might be arrested for practicing medicine without a license. This of course would hit the local newspapers and we found more practicing chiropractors becoming paranoid.

During the early part of the 20th-century, when the chiropractor's had anywhere from one year to 18 months of education, their diagnostic ability was limited. Their philosophy was, 'if the patients are breathing, adjust them'. This philosophy became more and more ignored with the fear of being arrested and possibly sued. Where the practitioners would roll up their sleeves and take any case it came in the door, the chiropractors in the 40's and 50's started referring more and more patience to the medical doctors. Instead of the state associations promoting positive results of chiropractic care they simply continued with administrative duties.

Many of the leaders in the profession, primarily those who lectured on clinical subjects and authors of research articles would continue to encourage the state associations to go on the offensive.

In the 1930's many chiropractors, in rural areas, were seeing over 100 patients per day. A medical spokesman told me a success rate of 35% was considered very well for the medical practitioner. I countered with the statement, that I could confirm, that a success rate of 85% to 93% was common for any chiropractor.

I had the opportunity to be on talk shows, both radio and television defending and advocating chiropractic care. I was always pared with a medical practitioner and in every case the chiropractic premise came out on top. This information, showing how the profession could stand its own ground was never disseminated to the profession to help instill pride within themselves.

In the latter half of the 20th-century the door was opened for advertisement in the phone books, on radio, on billboards and on television. By this time the profession of chiropractic had been readily recognized and accepted by the public. Unfortunately some wild claims were made by some practitioners, which only undermined the profession.

CHAPTER III

Schools

After 1911, with chiropractic growing in the Midwest, some type of legislative agreement had to be made since the chiropractic problem was not disappearing. In 1925 the state of Wisconsin passed a Workmen's Compensation law incorporating chiropractic care. It was the first in the country and gave the chiropractor's the opportunity to compile research and documentation. Unfortunately, this was not promoted by the state association or in any way enhanced by the schools.

The medical profession encouraged the Wisconsin legislators to pass a law requiring all graduates of medical, chiropractic, osteopathic and dental schools to pass the Basic Science exam before being examined by their own boards. It was assumed the chiropractors would fail to pass the examination, and therefore not be allowed to practice. In the ensuing years, the percentage of chiropractor's passing the examination far exceeded the medical doctors. When this became known, the examination was eliminated. Today of course, there are national boards for each profession along with State Board examinations. The professions are regulated by the Board of examiners who have complete jurisdiction over the particular profession.

In today's society, the chiropractor and medical doctor have the same education with four years of Pre-medical, Pre-chiropractic, and four years of graduate studies with the minimum of one-and-a-half years of internship. Education is not now nor ever was the problem facing the chiropractor. It was D.D. Palmer who stated "I can teach anyone to be a chiropractor in 30 days". That statement, before legislators, caused raised eyebrows because they did not understand the chiropractic philosophy of adjusting the spine to remove the cause of the malfunction.

The statement was made prior to 1910 and was brought up frequently during future legislative sessions.

Recognizing the early chiropractor's need to be accepted and free to practice without being arrested, we can see why research was not a priority. The chiropractor could not tell you why a simple adjustment of the vertebra from the sixth cervical to the second thoracic vertebrae would stop an asthma attack. Why an adjustment of the vertebra in the area of the fifth thoracic and eighth thoracic would reduce the effects of diabetes. Why an adjustment of the upper cervical spine would stop migraine headaches. His patients were not concerned why and the doctor wasn't either.

I met with leaders of the Muscular Dystrophy Association and suggested a research program utilizing chiropractic and medical practitioners. Success by individual chiropractors in caring for muscular dystrophy patients indicated a good possibility of success in reducing some of the effects of the condition. I was turned down regarding any future meeting. I met with the head of the Asthma Institute and suggested, with the success chiropractic had with reducing asthma attack a great step forward could be taken to relieve patients of this malady. Their recommendation was to implement a double blind study to show the effects of chiropractic and treatment of asthma. For a family practitioner, a double blind study is immoral, since it requires a patient to be treated without any hope of help by the use of a placebo.

My suggestion was to set up a clinic with both medical and chiropractic practitioners treating cases that had been evaluated by a committee of doctors to determine the effects of both treatments. Since medical doctors receive very little training in musculoskeletal diseases, this would provide a great step forward to relieve the suffering of millions by combining the best the two professions have to offer. This was also denied.

The chiropractic profession could easily, through its state associations, national associations, and colleges, provide such research. The opportunities wasted and bypassed from the 1930's, through 1970's is unfortunately a commentary of both professions. The medical profession, refusing to accept chiropractic research, and the chiropractic profession for not initiating such research.

Logan Basic Methods

The thinking, in the late 1800's and early 1900's, was centered on maintaining any healing procedure, passed down through the family, a secret. D.D. Palmer, upon 'discovering' a method to adjust the spinal vertebra, wanted this kept as a secret but his son, B.J. Palmer, saw the potential of the procedure and encouraged his father to start a school.

This thinking prevailed, unfortunately, into the late 20th-century. There is a story told about an early class at Palmer College where a previous graduate approached D.D. Palmer to point out he had found a way to adjust the vertebra at the base of the spine. He demonstrated by having a student lie on his side and bring his knee out into a flexed position. He then applied pressure to the knee, towards the floor and at the same time applied pressure to the shoulder on the same side causing the torso to twist. When he did this, there was a noticeable sound as the lower lumbar moved into position. With satisfaction on his face the returning student pointed out to Dr. Palmer he had just moved the fifth lumbar vertebra. Dr. Palmer's response was "no you just adjusted the first cervical with a different type of move". At that time, B.J. Palmer had advocated the adjustment of the first and second cervical vertebra were all that were necessary in the treatment of disease.

The returning student, according to the story, was Dr. Carver who went on to found the Carver Chiropractic College. Whether or not the story is true it does give the reader an understanding of the thinking of the times.

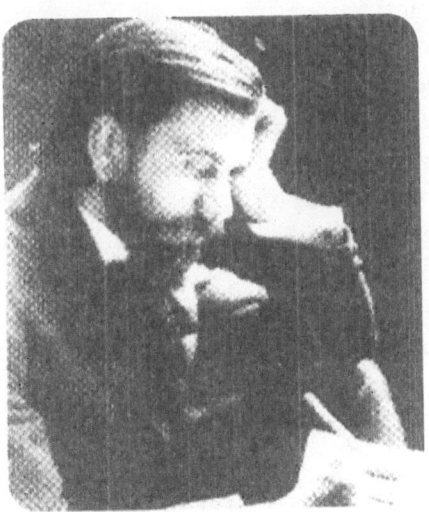

Dr. B. J. Palmer (Circa 1920))

In the late 1920's and early 30's, Dr. Hugh B. Logan, a graduate of universal chiropractic college, became concerned with the inability, particularly of the lower lumbar vertebra, to maintain stability after adjusting. His Research brought him the information on a non-force technique first applied by a medical doctor around 1906. Gathering some interested colleagues they began to research the effects of this technique and its proper application.

In the 1500's, publications depicted procedures for treating spinal curvatures, Scoliosis. No procedure in the last 400 years had been able to consistently and predictably reduce the curvature other than the application of surgery. Dr. Logan and his colleagues established the Logan system of body mechanics called Logan Basic Methods.

They established the IBTRI, the International Basic Technique Research Institute. It was to conduct research and to bring the information to field doctors, to help determine its validity. The response by the field doctors, to the weekend seminars, was sufficient to encourage Dr. Logan to open up a school in St. Louis Missouri to teach these procedures. It was the first clinical explanation of why vertebra will rotate in predictable sequence, measuring the rotation of the individual vertebra to determine the location of nerve impingement, and to produce a procedure by which a scoliosis, spinal curvature, could be reduced without braces and surgery.

The information, which concerned the greatest step forward in the practice of chiropractic since its inception, was ridiculed by the other colleges as a gimmick. Dr. Logan introduced full spine x-rays, full physical examinations and orthotics to the profession. He also established the first four-year graduate study for a doctor of chiropractic degree. This school began in 1935 and to this day is still, in the author's opinion, the premium school in the field of chiropractic. Having lectured on the Postgraduate faculty of nine other colleges, I feel qualified to make that statement.

If, (the most used word in the English language), the other colleges would have incorporated the information that Dr. Logan had researched, and set aside their personal agendas, the chiropractic profession would have grown in stature, respectability and acceptability by the academic community. I remember the president of one of the chiropractic colleges stating at a seminar that there was no other chiropractic college than his. With this myopic view of the world, it was a wonder the profession survived.

The Logan procedure enabled the doctor to determine physical conditions that had occurred earlier in life and to predict, with some accuracy, what conditions would appear later in life and then develop a procedure to forestall those conditions. It was one of the greatest breakthroughs in preventing malfunction at the time.

In the early 1900's the medical doctor prescribed medications to control symptoms. (Much the same as in the 21st century). The chiropractic profession had developed a procedure to determine the underlying cause of the symptom, and how to correct the causative factor. If the professions had joined together as a cohesive group, who knows how our health system would be today. This book is not written to provide solutions to our fouled up health care system but to give an opinion as to the events that precipitated the chiropractic profession's inability to move into the forefront of the health care providers.

Research has increased in the latter part of the 20th-century and has made some inroads into the cause and effect of spinal displacement. Dr. Suh, in the late 1980's, working at the University of Colorado on cadavers, determined that any displacement between two adjacent vertebrae of 4 mm or more will cause nerve impingement. This affirmation was first presented by Dr. Hugh B. Logan in the early 1930's when measurement of vertebra rotation was first taught in x-ray evaluation courses.

Clinical publications, in both clinical and scientific journals, by chiropractors, has increased in the last 30 years. The medical journals have been reluctant to except publications by chiropractors and once again, the inability of the medical profession to recognize the chiropractor's contribution to the health of the nation was apparent. Granted, no chiropractic research was carried on in the early part of the 20th-century as previously explained. With the muscular dystrophy telethon, accumulating $425 million, in a ten-year period, with no major results, imagine if thousands of chiropractor's were able to submit their data in the care of this condition. What results might have been found?

There were many other developments in the chiropractic profession during the first 50 years of the 20th-century. One of them was the neuro-colometer, developed by B.J. Palmer, which measured heat along the vertebral spine where a displacement of the vertebra might be found. The opportunity to provide this development with other schools did not present itself.

Most developments follow the course of specific procedures for adjusting vertebra and did little to increase the diagnostic ability of the average practitioner.

By the late 1920's many of the 117 chiropractic schools had passed by, and the stronger schools remained.

The techniques in themselves were very beneficial to the chiropractic profession but there was no major organization of chiropractic school administrators to correlate these findings to determine the professions effect on the population. Another factor, during this crucial time, was the insistence of the college leaders that their graduates only refer patients to fellow graduates. It was 'nationalism' that continued to separate the field practitioners. When district groups were formed in various states, to bring the chiropractors together, it was not unusual to see graduates of a particular school, congregate together. If one group achieved positions of leadership, in the district, there was dissension in the upper ranks.

It seems highly unusual what one considers all schools taught spinal bio mechanics, including procedures to adjust subluxated vertebrae and they still became divided based on procedures. While the medical doctors were advocating the use of medications and surgery for health-care the chiropractic profession was arguing over what areas should be adjusted and what technique should be used.

This is when, as an example, Palmer graduates would take over the leadership of the state association and impose their school philosophy. Graduates of other schools, all offended by this, started their own association. This has been mentioned before and why some states had as many as four state associations at one time.

Note:

I recently made my annual visit to the local Veterans Administration Clinic for my annual evaluation to remain in the VA system. The doctor, in his mid-40's, found out I was a retired chiropractor and started asking questions as to what it was like practicing over 50 years ago. He stated that the problem he had with his profession was not knowing if the medication he prescribed helped the patient or had the condition reached its climax. Were the efforts reduced, was there an emotional change in the patient, a stress release, or a change in the weather? The chiropractor, on the other hand, listened to their complaints, laid the patient down, placed their hands upon the patient and adjusted which vertebra they felt had a cause and effect concerning the condition. The patient left the office relieved of much of their discomfort.

He was familiar with the procedure having been to a chiropractor when he was younger and indicated many times that he wished the medical profession would be able to provide as much immediate relief to their patients as a chiropractor. He indicated "it's only getting worse with the continuing increase of medications that they are bombarded with on a daily basis". I pointed out my frustrations concerning the lack of cooperation between the professions which would have allowed the chiropractor to be the first entry point with the medical doctor providing what medications were designed to assist the body and its normal healing process. To paraphrase George Bernard Shaw's statement "England and America are two great countries separated by a common language", as, in my opinion, medicine and chiropractic are separated by an identical knowledge. You could also say chiropractors around the world are separated by a common philosophy.

Over the years, having had many opportunities to discuss medicine and chiropractic relationships with medical doctors, each one of them indicated they would not recommend medicine as a profession for their children. I must say, in all honesty, I never heard a chiropractor say they would not recommend chiropractic as a profession to their children, patients or friends.

CHAPTER IV

International Chiropractic Association
American Chiropractic Association

In 1926, it became apparent the chiropractic profession was growing at a terrific rate. Many of the schools, formed prior to and after World War I, were producing a goodly number of graduates. Many states did not recognize chiropractic and therefore there was no legislative control. What reasons B.J. Palmer had for starting the International Chiropractic Association are not clear. One would hope it would be to bring about long sought cohesion among the practitioners but events over the next 40 years prove this was not the primary intent. Considering the mentality of the individuals following World War I, it was possible most professional advancements were redirected towards personal recognition. The individuals chosen to run the I.C.A. were of course, Palmer college graduates. The designation 'straight chiropractor's' surface itself to denote those individuals utilizing spinal adjustment only in their practice. The late 1920's saw the growth of many modalities that chiropractors were eager to purchase to add to their modus operandi. Many of them were not proficient at spinal adjustment and without licensing laws, there was no way to test the doctor's ability. I do firmly believe there is nothing new under the sun and that the Lord provides inspiration for the betterment of mankind. The philosophy of chiropractic is simple and to the point. The application of chiropractic is also simple and to the point but unfortunately the results of chiropractic treatment are many times better than the applicator that provided the adjustment. The I.C.A. continued to promote spinal adjusting by hand rather than use various modalities. It was the doctors who lacked the confidence in their adjusting procedures who procured most of the modalities and caused a further split in the profession.

By 2008, the I.C.A. office indicates they have 4,454 members. They indicate there are 51,000 practicing chiropractors. The I.C.A. has been very active on the legislative front of every state where chiropractic legislation has been introduced. According to the record, as of today, they represent less than 10% of the practicing chiropractors. In 1955 the colleges estimated there were 50,000 practicing chiropractors. Based on those figures the profession has not grown in over 50 years. It is also estimated in 2008 there are 10,000 students in the 17 colleges in the United States.

American Chiropractic Association

By the end of World War Two, the influx of students into chiropractic colleges was very noticeable, as veterans returned to start their careers. The changes manifested by the returning veterans, upset with the state of the status quo and their willingness to insert new ideas, and started a wave of change within the chiropractic profession. In 1963 the American Chiropractic Association was formed. One would imagine the I.C.A., having been around for 40 years would be the magnet drawing all chiropractors into its fold. The old guard was very evident in all deliberations concerning legislative licensing of chiropractors. The A.C.A. advocated a much more liberal (medically orientated) practice within the profession. By 2008, the American Chiropractic Association claims 16,000 members out of a projected population of 60,000 practicing chiropractors, less than 30%. Both organizations combined comprise less than 30% of the profession.

The opportunity for Chiropractic to move into the forefront of the health-care system was once again lost in 1926 with the self-serving attitude of the I.C.A. and 1963 when the I.C.A. and A.C.A. could not, for the betterment of mankind, combine their forces to rise up and provide research, education and information to the population.

There were more battles in the legislative halls of states between the A.C.A and I.C.A. as to the inclusions in legislative bills. There was opposition by the AMA. In testifying before the state Senate, and Committee Chairman, I became very much aware of the strong belief differences among chiropractors. It seems they had, as a profession, reconciled themselves, since the early years, to be second-class health-care providers and therefore felt it was more important for them to maintain their personal beliefs that may differ from their colleagues, than to unify and to demand their rightful place in the health-care system.

In the latter half of the 20th-century, more advanced training was provided the chiropractic profession on the Postgraduate level. Graduate school, for both the chiropractor and a medical doctor, primarily provides them with the knowledge to pass the national boards. Postgraduate internship and resident training teaches the specialties. The A.C.A. began setting up divisions in the organization to deal with the specialties. The specialties included radiology, neurology, nutrition, sports chiropractic and others. Having been a charter member of the A.C.A., I was involved in the early meetings dealing with specialties. With the A.C.A. and I.C.A., being so far apart on their philosophical level, it was impossible to get proper recognition from state legislative bodies to recognize these specialties. As a licensed practitioner, I decided to re-enter the Army after graduation. I was told by the army my graduate degree and state license would allow me to empty the bedpans, at the rank of private. The two professional organizations in chiropractic were unable to provide a united front to the United States Senate to allow graduate chiropractors an equal position with the medical profession in the armed forces.

This lost opportunity was not offset by the identification of chiropractic in the insurance industry, Medicare and Medicaid.

When the U. S. Senate considered including chiropractic into Medicare and Medicaid the same old battle was renewed. I had heard testimony by the medical profession that there was no such thing as a vertebral subluxation. Both professions study from the same books dealing with anatomy, neurology, osteology and histology, all of which confirmed the displacement of vertebral segments. (Subluxations)

When it became apparent the Senate was going to agree to include chiropractic in Medicare and Medicaid, the A.M.A. representative assured the Senate committee, that in order to protect the lay population from quackery, all Medicare patients going to a chiropractor must be X-rayed by the chiropractor without renumeration. Each X-ray must be sent to a medical doctor to determine if a subluxation exists. Before we could treat a patient, the medical doctor had to confirm there was a subluxation, which they did not believe existed. The chiropractic representatives, like a donkey following a carrot on a stick, grabbed at the carrot rather than stand up for their equal rights as state licensed practitioners. At this time, the Senate already agreed to allow veterans to attend chiropractic colleges under the G I Bill. For many years the chiropractor's were subjected to the embarrassing process of having to charge patients for X-rays, without reimbursement by Medicare and then wait for a medical doctor to say yes there is a subluxation and then allow the chiropractor 10 treatments within a 12 month period. It is interesting to note the patient with an arthritic spine and disk degeneration may be X-rayed by the medical doctor 'prescribed medications' and receive daily treatment as long as the medical doctor deems necessary. The chiropractor accepting the same patient must charge them for the film's, treat them no more than 10 times and receive payment at a rate up to 20% under what it costs to provide the care.

If our national organizations had combined sufficiently with the state organizations and stood up for their rights, the profession would have had to except the crumbs it received. It has been over 40 years since the United States government had been petitioned to allow chiropractors to be at the same level of acceptance in the armed forces as the medical doctors and still nothing has been accomplished.

It is understood, as previously mentioned, that with out control over the individual chiropractor, and the scope of practice, it is almost impossible to police the profession to eliminate the bad apples. Not that the medical profession as been able to clear their bad apples, even with their control.

It may be a change in the times that the young doctors of today, regardless of their profession, do not like to be controlled. My understanding, from the A.M.A. is their membership, in relation to the number practicing medical doctors, has reduced over the last few decades.

Around the middle of the 20th-century there were letter-writing campaigns, phone contacts and concentrated efforts to bring about legislative acceptance on the state level but never substantially on the national level. Today we set with two national organizations comprising less the 30% of the population a practicing chiropractic doing very little to bring about changes that should have been done 50 years ago.

In the 1970's a survey conducted in the state of Wisconsin indicated the average chiropractor saw 100 new patients per year that had never previously been a chiropractic patient. At that time there were over 1000 chiropractor's practicing in Wisconsin. That implied there were 100,000 people exposed to chiropractic in one-year and with the 80+% success rate in relieving pain and suffering in a few short visits, the medical profession was highly concerned about the economics of allowing chiropractor's more freedom of practice. This became very evident in the Senate committee hearings and I am sure manifested itself on the national level.

World Posture Queen Pageant

In the late 1940's, Dr. Clair O'Dell of Michigan, formed the World Posture Queen Pageant to bring chiropractic to the public. He worked directly with Logan College of Chiropractic in St. Louis to help establish the pageant. It was his intention, since pageants were very common promotional ideas at the time, to make the population aware of the benefits of a straight spine and healthy body. Each district, in a state, would compete to have a young woman with a straight spine and healthy body be crowned Posture Queen of that state. Each state would compete at the World Posture Queen Pageant. The pageants were held in such cities as Montreal Canada, St Louis Missouri Chattanooga Tennessee, Loss Angeles California and San Juan P.R. It accomplished what Dr. O'Dell wanted which included television coverage of the pageant, radio and television interviews of the contestants and news coverage. The public relations this received was monumental since prior to this time no Chiropractic activity had been on prime time news broadcasts and front-page coverage. Unfortunately, neither national organization provided full support. By the 1970's the pageant had brought awareness to much of the country and was discontinued. Sometimes playing catch-up is just too tiring.

Having had the opportunity to be interviewed on both television and radio when the pageants were presented in different cities, we contacted the state associations to let them know we would be in their state in order to promote chiropractic. Recognizing the necessity for public awareness of what chiropractic provides it seemed ridiculous some state associations decided not to offer local support or to follow-up the pageant with their own public relations. This was a new venture in the late 1940's and 50's whose mission was to help the population understand that not only is the chiropractor similarly educated as the medical profession but licensed as one of only three professions licensed to treat the patient from dandruff to athlete's foot. Many times in discussions with individuals who had graduated in the 20's and early 30's it became apparent why the profession was unable to gain proper recognition. It did not deal with education even though the lay population had been bombarded with the understanding that the medical doctors eight years of college, year of internship plus residency made them the only ones capable of determining what type of health-care could be presented to the population.

The pageant, through interviews, provided the listener and viewer to understand that the chiropractor upon graduation and finishing their internship were fully capable of providing proper health care based on their philosophy and training. The medical profession, due to the development of specialties and the influence the leaders in those specialties provided the hospitals to develop a system where in the specialty was protected from the infusion of someone outside that specialty. I have been on hospital staffs and privy to many behind-the-scenes conversations and observed how an ob/gyn would not be allowed to remove an appendix because that infringed upon the general surgeon's area. This established more of a selective hierarchy requiring the patient to be transferred from one specialty to another. Not denying the value of the specialties but it did remove the family doctor from the availability to the population. No longer could your family doctor deliver your baby, take out your tonsils, set your broken arm or spend the night at your side. Advancements are necessary but the chiropractic profession, comfortable in their area of quick results neglected to inform the population of their existence. I made daily house calls, as did most of my colleagues, for almost 50 years. The patients recognized this personal care by my colleagues and me. The state associations, even after hiring public relations firms did not project the picture of the concerned doctor of chiropractic standing at the bedside in the middle of the night providing comfort to the patient. The only movie picture available during the 1960's concerning chiropractic was 'Come Back Little Sheba', a story about a drunken chiropractor.

Having lectured and taught both chiropractors and medical doctors, the biggest complaints I heard from chiropractic was "If I have one more patient say to me, 'You don't treat children do you?' I think I will blow my mind". Chiropractors have been classed as doctors who treat backaches. Over 30 percent of my practice was children, the same for most other practitioners. Our range of ages in patients ran from the new born to centurions. There are many stories that can be told about 'miracles' performed by chiropractors on house calls during the last 100 years. The purpose of this writing, as previously stated, is to inform the reader of how a profession gifted with the ability to remove pain and suffering was delegated to second-class citizenship. It's not sour grapes but simply answering the question, if chiropractic is so good why hasn't it achieved a higher standing in the health-care system?

Specialties

Chiropractic specialties are developed on an individual basis primarily by doctors, who by research and daily application of a technique, determined that that particular procedure was outside the mainstream of those practicing chiropractic. We must remember the chiropractor in the first 40 years of the 20th-century was instructed solely to adjust mis-aligned vertebra. Other than some diagnostic procedures advocated by the colleges, every chiropractor did the same thing to their patients varied only in the amount of force and application that they would provide. There were seven ways to adjust a vertebra, the same direction, so each doctor used the procedure based on there dexterity.

Dr. Grostic was one of the first to advocate adjusting only the cervical spine based on some information that B.J. Palmer had advocated. It became the Grostic procedure and to this day is practiced by some individuals. This specialty is an accepted procedure but the national organizations never utilized the media to indicate to the public that this was an accepted procedure. Many patients would be told by their doctor if they ever needed to find a practitioner in another community they would only go to those who graduated from the same college. This is not an unusual approach since certain ailments could require individuals trained in application of specific techniques. Another practitioner by the name of Nimo developed a trigger point procedure in the 1930's preceding the introduction of the field of Meridian Therapy by almost 70 years. The procedure, extremely valuable, was not accepted by the National Associations for research and therefore was not presented to the public.

The development of Logan Basic Technique and the formation of Logan College in 1935 was the first in formalizing a technique with an educational institution. The non-force technique had been proven to provide specific reduction in cases of spinal curvatures, known as scoliosis. At the time of its establishment, the only national organizations were the I.C.A. and N.C.A. They specifically limited all treatment to adjustments of the spine by manual application. The I.C.A. in its inevitable wisdom, discounted the procedures to the extent of informing students it was a fraud. I personally had attended lectures by the I.C.A. where this was said.

Those of us on lecture circuits dealing with clinical subjects have a totally different outlook and understanding of techniques. As with religion, we can become tolerant of the other fellow as long as they do no harm and provide for the patients welfare. Unfortunately, there are the 'snake oil salesmen' who stick their heads up periodically and come up with a procedure or technique that, to them, is divinely inspired and the salvation of all mankind. The presentation is to the chiropractic profession and because not all doctors graduate at the top of their class and many who pass the boards do not have the dexterity to be good adjusters and become prime believers in procedures that are really a 'pie in the sky' dream.

The national organizations miss the opportunity when fund raising marathons were first thought of by the A.M.A. to fund research. Therefore, with the I.C.A. being the only national organization in the chiropractic profession up until 1963, it was either my way or the highway. When fund raising was in its infancy it would have been easy for the profession to start a grass roots wave of support for specific education of the population.

It would have been a simple procedure to have every practicing chiropractor work with their patients to set up fund-raising for research. In 1976 I proposed establishing a free clinic for the treatment of scoliosis by chiropractors. Plans were drawn up for a facility about one hundred thousand square feet utilizing ample documentation to treat a condition that had been identified in the Middle Ages. Because the recognized procedures to be used did not have the endorsement of the I.C.A or A.C.A., it never got off the ground. Doctors were asked to donate one afternoon a week to work in the facility. The chiropractic profession had never been encouraged to develop research programs or to volunteer their time and talents for that type of cause. The promotional attitude seemed to be 'each man is an island'. The facility never got off the ground since even the state association would not utilize their public-relations firm to promote such a facility.

Another example of the mentality promoted by the state association's happened when it was decided to establish a chiropractic office in the black community in Milwaukee Wisconsin. There were no black chiropractors in the black community and they never had the profession brought into their culture. It was determined an office would be opened and young black women would be trained as office help in the areas of accounting, doctor assistants, X-ray technicians and insurance clerks. The leaders in the black community were simply asked to provide a facility in which this free clinic could operate. They refused primarily because they didn't even know what a chiropractor was. With the advent of television, fund-raising reached a new high and had the opportunity to bring to the public information concerning the chiropractic profession, its history, its education and its effect upon the health of the nation.

The A.C.A. began to recognize specialties and set up councils within the organization. They established radiology, nutrition, orthopedics and other councils. Not for the purpose of bringing this information to the public but actually for a purpose that no one knows. Possibly for self-edification.

It is interesting that after 55 years of being a chiropractor, people still ask "do you treat headaches? do you treat stomach problems? to you treat children?"

How can a profession that has been in existence as a health-care provider for 108 years still have a majority of the population not having any understanding of what care they provide. Granted they are licensed in all 50 states, have colleges in six different countries and treat, conservatively, over 1 million patients per month. As one individual said "it is the world's best kept secret", other than Christianity.

The demise of the chiropractic profession comes about, in my opinion, as the full fault of the national organizations with their myopic leadership, un-willing to promote all aspects of the profession, that provides their livelihood.

Publications

The first half of the 20th-century found the individual chiropractor functioning in their own world, observing unbelievable results in the relief of pain and suffering. This only seemed to isolate them more and more as individuals and other than some socializing and state association meetings there was not enough of interchange of ideas. As with medical doctors, when they find a specific medication that works for certain conditions, it is difficult for them to change to something else, same as with surgical procedures.

Towards the middle of the 20th-century publications began to appear. The most noticeable were Chiropractic Economics, American Chiropractor, Today's Chiropractic and MPI out of California from the Motion Palpation Institute. The publications, besides providing advertisements for various supplements and equipment, did encourage doctors to provide case studies for publication. This then produced clinical articles based on the doctor's individual recognition of certain treatment procedures and the results.

Clinical articles do not carry any credibility in the scientific community but do provide information to the reader as to the acceptability of the procedure described by the case study.

The National College of Chiropractic in Lombard Illinois, published the first indexed Journal, in the chiropractic profession and was accepted by the scientific community. The editorial board was made up of practicing chiropractor's, which manifested, once again, the individual chiropractor's school philosophy.

As an example of narrow thinking taught by some schools, I submitted a research paper to the chiropractic-indexed journal concerning the treatment protocols for spinal scoliosis. Sixty-eight cases were drawn randomly from hundreds of recorded cases. The article contained charts and results based on a one-year control period. The article indicated positive results in reduction of the scoliosis in every one of the 68 cases. Since the procedure used was only taught at Logan College, the doctors on the editorial board felt it was not possible to get 100% response based on the education they received and they denied the right to publish the report.

Once again, the lack of acceptance by schools and the national organizations to disseminate legitimate, clinically proven procedures to solidify the profession became evident. As one Academic Dean explained to me when I provided a Postgraduate clinical seminar, "if we don't teach it, it doesn't exist".

I was informed by medical writers that they received financial renumeration when articles were submitted to their publication. The chiropractic publications also accepted clinical articles from doctors who wished to publish. Unfortunately, there is no compensation from chiropractic journals. Therefore, the incentive to compile the facts necessary to publish a clinically correct article may end up being about the doctor's un-substantiated belief, for self-edification. This then did not allow for a true control of what was printed. When one is paid to write an article they are establishing a reputation based on the information there providing and, in my opinion, are far more stringent in the facts they provide. The others many times just like to see their name in print.

One of the offsets in developing publications for the profession was the infusion of Practice Management organizations. The medical and chiropractic colleges had not provided the students with basic business courses to run the office or clinic. The practice management people saw this as a golden opportunity and quickly moved to convince the doctors how to run an office. Many doctors, who were not confident and outgoing, jumped at the opportunity to provide these practice management people with the percentage of their income because they were promised they could become millionaires. The basic philosophy of a doctor is to relieve suffering and do no harm. Practice management people, with full-page ads and promises which could not be fulfilled, encourage the young doctors to develop an economic philosophy. Some of them became very successful and became millionaires, but the profession suffered from its lost ideology. The patients became numbers at office visits were many times reduced to less than two minutes. The publications were in business to make money so it was not their responsibility to regulate the profession. However, I do feel both the schools and associations did little to direct the doctors back to their oath. It was not unusual to have a lecture hall with twenty-five doctors learning new treatment techniques next to an auditorium with five hundred doctors learning how to make more money.

In the 1970's the chiropractic Editors Guild was formed involving editors of all the state journals. The purpose was to standardize the publications that, at the time, varied from one page mimeographed sheets, 4-5 page newspapers and professionally done publications. The state associations, responsible for these publications, simply ask for volunteers to put them together. The volunteers were doctors, most of whom had no background putting together a journal. The Editors organization was in effect for ten years but since the state associations kept changing the editors of their publications, based on who volunteered, eventually most publications stopped being distributed. Once again no support on a state or national level. Both the I.C.A. and A.C.A. had their publications but limited the publication of articles to members only.

In the 1980's I had the honor of being chosen to be a member of an editorial board of one of the national magazines. The magazine had a fine reputation and was a quality publication. I was never quite sure about the percentage allocated for clinical articles vs. practice management articles but did seem to find, if one includes the full-page advertisements, a higher percentage of promotional type articles than those based on clinical subjects was evident. The editorial board did work to balance this presentation while recognizing that practice management articles were in direct relationship to the advertising they purchased, which keeps the magazine alive. The owners of the magazine did continue to add more and more clinical data including specific monthly articles on subjects such as X-ray procedures, nutrition, sports chiropractic and many other subjects. The magazine is still one of the top publications but, like many, is on a subscription basis and therefore not reaching the full population of chiropractor's. The discussion continues to be about the simple statement 'chiropractic treatment provides such a high percentage of results in a short period of time, the practicing chiropractor does not feel the need to study extensively'. Doctors, who specialize in the various aspects of chiropractic, do utilize publications and seminars, but the percentage of specializing chiropractors is small compared to the full population of practitioners.

CHAPTER V

Curriculum & Missed Opportunities

In the early part of the 20th-century, basic rudiments in chiropractic college curriculums dealt with the specific art of adjusting vertebra. As previously mentioned there are seven ways to move any one vertebra the same way. What this implies is that, any vertebra may move in many rotational positions, such as rotate right, rotate left, tip the vertebra superior or inferior, posterior or anterior. There is also the combination of any two or more of these positions. Each move was designated by the vertebral position, such as an anterior, posterior or rotational move to the right or left. The contact point, on the vertebra was also used as a description of the type of move, such as a lamina, spinous transverse move. The size of the doctor's hand, combined with their dexterity, determined the type of move they may use in the adjustment of a vertebra. The variation in dexterity separated the very good adjusters from the poor. This was the reason many chiropractors adapted to use various modalities and instrumentation to provide their treatment protocols. I have visited offices where the patient was first provided with hydroculator treatment, (hot or cold packs), then put on a traction machine, followed by muscle stem or ultrasound. The patient rarely received a vertebral adjustment because the chiropractor was not confident in their ability to perform the proper adjustment. Therefore, the chiropractor applied a variety of ancillary procedures and felt justified in charging the patient for chiropractic care. As with the medical doctors today, based on the American Medical Association survey in 2008, 50 percent of internists prescribe placebos for patients, without informing the patients that the prescription they are receiving has absolutely nothing to do with the complaint that they presented to the doctor. This procedure maintains their role, as a physician, even though they have no idea how to treat the problem.

The curriculum provided by the colleges of chiropractic has been increased since the first quarter of the 20th-century. As the doctors were taught anatomy and other clinical subjects, the school term was lengthened. By the mid-1930's, Logan College started the first four-year curriculum. Since most college and universities have a nine-month school year, the chiropractic colleges did a 12-month school year for three years. Residency requirements call for 36 months in the medical field. This can be done in four years of nine months each year or three years of 12 months each year. The subjects that were added, by Logan College, far exceeded those subjects offered by other colleges, with the addition of histology, osteology, embryology, pathology, differential diagnosis, two years of anatomy, and a year of radiology.

Note:

In 1953 I received 300 hours in the study of roenconolgy, (x-ray), while the medical schools in Wisconsin were not providing the medical doctor with any instruction in the field of X-ray. It was in effect, an extra curricular subject. The medical doctors I had met, during my years in practice, could not read X-rays and had to rely on the new specialty in the medical profession called radiologists. There were many occasions when I had to explain to a medical doctor what was seen on the film.

The number of classroom hours required in 1953 to obtain a medical license in the state of Wisconsin was 4200. When I graduated, Logan College required 4400 classroom hours, plus 18 months of internship in outpatient clinics. The medical doctor, after finishing his graduate studies, did an internship in various local hospitals. Then moves on to a residency in the specialty they wish to follow. The chiropractic student, after finishing their 18 months of supervised internship in out patient clinics may decide to learn one of the specialties available to Postgraduate studies offered by the colleges.

Both the chiropractic and a medical graduate were required the 1950's and 60's to take what was known as the Basic Science examination in the state of Wisconsin. The chiropractor, medical doctor, osteopath and dentist all took the same examination. If they passed this examination they were then sent on to their individual board for further examination to obtain a license to practice in the state.

Over the years it was interesting to note the medical profession continually promoted the idea the chiropractor was un-educated by having only three months of schooling. This of course was totally inaccurate and as I pointed out, when I was spokesman for the Wisconsin Chiropractic Association, speaking on NBC, if we all the had three months of education why were more chiropractor's passing the Basic Science examination, on a per-capita basis, than the medical doctors. Since the chiropractor's were passing the examination it was determined in the second half of the 20th century to eliminate the Basic Science examination and each of the professions then formed national boards to precede any State Board examinations. The Basic Science was initially presented to the state legislature, in the 1920's, by the Medical Society of Wisconsin, in order to prevent chiropractor's from obtaining a license. In the beginning of the formation of the Basic Science examination they had a separate section called 'Special on the Spine'. In the promotion of the Basic Science examination it was stated that it is impartial and it no one would know who had taken examination. The problem with that was that only a chiropractor would take the Spine Special and it is interesting to note the failure rate of the Spine Special examination far exceeded the failure rate of the chiropractor's taking the standard Basic Science examination.

When I took the examination in 1953 at Marquette University in Milwaukee Wisconsin the exam was taken in an auditorium with the four professions, medical, chiropractic, osteopathic and dental. I sat in a group of medical students and the one sitting next to me said "This is a waste of time for me since I will never pass the examination". When I asked why, since he had finished four years of school, he said "I got in trouble mouthing off to the head bigwigs at school and I know I was put on their list and I know they will fail me".

The state association had every opportunity to bring awareness to the public of the chiropractor's educational background and licensing procedures but nothing was ever done by the Wisconsin Chiropractic Association. Neither the National Organization nor the College Presidents Association ever combined efforts to inform the public of the chiropractor's educational background and requirements.

Medically we were referred to as bone crackers and cultists. Of course, the medical profession had been referred to as 'sawbones' and other phrases, but as an underdog profession it was hard for the chiropractor's to provide help when needed when they were referred to as uneducated.

As mentioned before, specialties within the chiropractic profession became noticeable in the 1970's. The American chiropractic Association recognized certain specialties within their own membership and would not recognize any other specialties. The International Chiropractic Association did not recognize those specialties endorsed by A.C.A. and consequently the public was left un-aware of this advanced education available by some practicing chiropractors.

Patients would enter our office after not receiving any relief from their problem with their family doctor. If after a few chiropractic treatments they received relief, they would say "I cannot tell my family doctor that you did relieve me of my problem because he would get mad. I told him I might go to a chiropractor and he said you may end up dying from a broken neck or broken back". The lack of education of the public was also transferred to the medical profession. I had personal friends in the medical profession who told me they were taught in school that chiropractor's were un-educated charlton's and quacks and that it is unethical for them to associate socially or professionally with cultists. The fact was brought to my attention when a medical doctor wanted to rent office space from me in one of the buildings I owned. We had consummated the deal when the doctor called and said "I must notify the state association of our address. When they ask her who the others were in the building and she told them a chiropractor they said she would not be able to keep her hospital Association credentials if she was in the same office building with a chiropractor". Therefore, the lease was canceled.

COUNCIL ON CHIROPRACTIC EDUCATION

The following information is taken from the web site of the Council on Chiropractic Education. The information presented on the Web site disagrees with some historians concerning specific dates. The information is relevant since it does show the chiropractic profession was interested in increasing the educational standards of the profession. Yet information presented, is not word for word but does cover the highlights of the formation of the Council on Chiropractic education.

Note: From the web page:

In the development of the Council on Chiropractic Education, the importance of quality education was recognized early in the chiropractic profession. Voluntary efforts to improve chiropractic education were undertaken as early as 1935 when the National Chiropractic Association, (N.C.A.) created a committee on educational standards. During the years between 1935 and 1940 various national chiropractic associations such as the N.C.A., Chiropractic Health Bureau, and the Council on State Chiropractic Examining Boards supported the improvement of chiropractic education with both funds and human power. Years later, the N.C.A became the American Chiropractic Association and the Chiropractic Health Bureau became the International Chiropractors Association (I.C.A.)

In 1938 the first institution of self-study questionnaire was sent to all 37 chiropractic institutions actively engaged in chiropractic education in the United States.

In 1939 C.B.S. completed work on educational criteria, which were presented for approval of the chiropractic institutions. In 1947 institutional representatives and members of the C.B.S. formed the Council on education. On August 4th 1947 this council received the approval and support of the House of Delegates of the N.C.A. In 1952 the Council on Education made the initial contact with the United States Office of Education, later to become the United States Department of Education. From 1941 to 1961 the council continued to strengthen chiropractic education. Many of the weaker institutions were merged with other institutions to create stronger academic positions. A number of the institutions were closed. By 1961 the number of institutions had been reduced to 10.

In 1964 the N.C.A. merged with other groups to form the A.C.A., (American Chiropractic Association), which continues to implement, and support the council on education. Suggestions for strengthening academics and procedures were received and implemented, and in 1969 and un-official filing of materials with the United States Department of Education resulted in further suggestions for change. In 1971 the Council on Chiropractic Education was incorporated as an autonomous national organization and continues to this day.

On August 16, 1972, C.C.E. filed a formal application and on August 26th 1974, the U.S. Commissioner of Education from the Department of Health Education and Welfare first answered the accrediting commission of the recognized accrediting agency as an association for a period of one year.

C.C.E. was accepted as a member of the council in 1975. in December of 1975 the commissioner extended the period for three years.

On July 1, 1976 The New York State legislative body accepted the criteria of C.C.E. to be able to license chiropractors in their state. (End of the Web page information)

The Council on Chiropractic Education filled a very great space within the profession. Before the formation of C.C.E., individual schools set up their curriculum, established school hours, set up clinical criteria and determined length of the residency. The C.C.E. in getting acceptance by the United States Department of Education had the authority to withdraw certification from any school that did not adhere to the standards established by C.C.E.. Some schools received a three-year acceptance when others, due to their discrepancies, received only one year of acceptance. When the school loses its C.C.E. acceptance, the graduates of that college are not allowed to take either the National Board or the State Board examinations for a license. It was a necessary move, upon the profession, to obtain this accreditation. As of this day, there are seventeen accredited colleges, in the United States. There are also colleges in Canada, Japan, South Africa, Australia and England. The French medical society was successful in closing the chiropractic college in Paris France.

Unfortunately, the National Board's, in conducting their examinations, of which there are three, still do not encompass the chiropractic philosophy in their examinations but lean heavily upon medical clinical evaluation. Example: Logan College has taught, both in their graduate and postgraduate courses, the clinical proven procedures for the reduction of spinal Scoliosis by chiropractic procedures. The National Board continues to require medical interpretation for the treatment of scoliosis which requires referring all cases of 20-degree curvature or more to an orthopedic surgeon. My personal discussions with those in charge of the examinations accomplished nothing. There are too many pseudo medical doctors in positions of power in the chiropractic profession. They enjoy the right to be called doctor, the right to wear the stethoscope around their necks and like to wear surgical scrubs in their office. The graduates of certain schools are informed by their schools, that other chiropractic colleges are not teaching the proper chiropractic philosophy according to their interpretation.

This was to be carried to an extreme when graduates of certain schools were placed in complete charge of State Board licensing examinations. An example would be the chiropractic Board of Examiners in the state of Wisconsin in the 1950's. The Palmer chiropractic college graduates were considered 'straight' chiropractor's, which meant that they adjust the spine by hand without the use of any modalities. They were informed, by their school, that any other college would be considered 'mixers', because they not only utilized medical diagnosis but involve themselves with ancillary types of treatment. Division, in the profession, became so strong that another organization was formed within the state of Wisconsin, called the Wisconsin Chiropractic Society. Palmer College graduates, in charge of the Board of Examiners, did what they could to limit granting licenses to the mixers.

Having had four doctors working for me, in my clinic and having them represent three specific colleges, with different philosophies, proved to be a problem when filing insurance forms. Since the 'straight' chiropractor did not believe in physical examinations and the 'mixer' wanted to send the patients to the hospital for a blood tests, it was necessary to eliminate some of the doctors in order to maintain the unified approach to proper practice.

Chiropractic colleges were privately funded, deriving much of their income from their outpatient clinics and student tuition. Unlike the medical schools, who as part of the state university system was supported by state funds, grants and federal assistance. Because each chiropractic college was in direct competition with other chiropractic colleges and were unable to receive state or federal funds, some of the school leaders took upon themselves to downgrade every other college, but their own, to maintain a steady influx of students.

I listened to the head of the International Chiropractic Association tell me that the only college teaching chiropractic principles was Palmer college and all other colleges were frauds. This attitude permeated the chiropractic profession for the first half of the 20th-century. The seeds were planted in those early years for the future demise of the chiropractic profession as the leading health care system available to the population.

Today, the country has a major problem with our health-care system. The medical profession is not part of the health-care system, but a part of the 'disease' care system. Their main treatment and orientation is the treatment of disease and elimination of symptoms through the use of medications. The chiropractic profession maintains its position in the health-care system by restoring the body's natural function to prevent the inception of disease.

The inability of the I.C.A. and A.C.A. to bring the schools into unification as a unified force in presenting chiropractic philosophy and care to the population, continued to undermine the professions credibility.

A very simple solution, to what is considered our national 'health-care' problem would be to form a 'Triage' in every hospital made up of representatives of each medical specialty and chiropractors. When a patient is admitted the panel determines which patients need immediate emergency care and others are turned over to the chiropractors to determine if their condition can be improved in 72 hours by the use of medications to control pain, and chiropractic care to restore the body to natural function. This, of course can never happen, since chiropractors have not been able to assume any similar position in a tax supported hospital. Any qualified chiropractor could reduce hospital admissions by 36%. This could never be accepted by the medical community. Having been in the same area for forty-seven years, I was frequently called to the hospital, by my patients when the medical doctors could not provide help.

I know this sounds unfamiliar to the unacquainted but I will sight just two cases to give you an indication of why I feel the chiropractic profession missed its calling to provide care to the population.

The first case involved a young woman in her 20's, who had been a polio victim at age 12 which left her paralyzed at the lower extremities. I had been providing her chiropractic care for six years during which she had developed increase mobility, was able to become a receptionist at a doctor's office and became more independent.

She developed a vomitting attack, which frightened her parents and caused them to call their family doctor who admitted her to the local hospital. three days later, she still could not raise her head off the pillow without regurgitating. They called me and asked if I would come to the hospital and help her. We asked the nurse to leave the room and moving the bed away from the wall I adjusted the cervical vertebra. She sat up in bed, free of nausea and had no more regurgitation. Her family doctor indicated it was obviously a spontaneous remission and she could go home. The family told me later that they had asked their family doctor if I could come and provide her with care and he vehemently protested.

Another case was one that made the front page of the local paper. A young man, in his late teens had been suffering convulsions, up to 15 times a day. Specialists had been brought in, when he was admitted to the hospital, and they were unable to determine the diagnosis. For two or three days, the paper carried daily reports on his condition. Canisters were setup in local businesses to raise money for his care. After one week, I contacted the family and offered my services, since the last report indicated the parents had been told nothing could be done and that he may suffer a fatal heart attack during a convulsion. I made daily house calls for three weeks. At the end of that time, he had between two and three convulsions a week and they were mild. When the family reported this to the reporters at the paper, the published article indicated he had mysteriously improved when he was sent home.

These are two of many cases taking place over the years that, in my opinion, confirm the fact that the average chiropractor could well reduce the number of patients in hospitals, if provided access.

CHAPTER VI

Politics—subsidizing professionals
Sponsoring political candidates

Politics and chiropractic did not become integrated, to any degree, until after World War II. It wasn't until 1935 in the state of Wisconsin that dentists were allowed to be called doctors by the state legislature. Chiropractors had fought long and hard to have their degree recognized so they too could be referred to as doctors.

The politicians had long understood the chiropractic profession was not only disorganized but also incapable of getting their memberships to agree on any legislative proposal. It wasn't until both state organizations combined to form a unified front that they were able to present legislative proposals that could be accepted. During the period from 1960 through 1980 much legislation was passed including the requirement for all insurance companies to include chiropractic care, along with Medicare and Medicaid. The Veterans Administration, to this day, does not provide chiropractic care for veterans.

When I served on the board of the Wisconsin Chiropractic Association, I had opportunities to testify before the state Senate, and to meet with Committee Chairman, both in the capital and in the local restaurants where most of the politicking took place. I remember one specific state senator who commented to me over lunch, "I see the chiropractors have finally arrived on the scene". When I asked him how this was determined, he said "You now know who to slip the money to". It was true we had been contacted by Committee Chairman and told that if you want a bill out of committee, compensation must be made available. We had arrived !

One of the bills we had worked on for three years was passed and sent to the governor for his signature. I was privileged to be at his desk when he signed the bill. One year later, we had found the bill had not been implemented, and began an investigation to find out why. We discovered a department head had put the signed bill in his desk drawer and did not release it because he didn't like chiropractors. Fortunately, this only happened one time and we were able to pass beneficial legislation for the public. One of the more important aspects of our successful approach to the state legislators was the formation of a telephone network. We had a committee going over every bill submitted to the legislature. The State Medical Society included amendments restricting chiropractic every time they could, in bills that seemed to have no reference to health care. When the committee would discover these amendments, calls would be made to individual chiropractors, who in turn would call others until hundreds of chiropractor's would call their senator or representative to give them an opinion. Many times when the bill was introduced, the legislator would be overcome by the number of messages on their phone from their constituents.

From the beginning, feelings ran very hot between the mixers and straights. The same feelings ran high no matter how beneficial legislation would be both to the public and chiropractic. Individual chiropractors would take-off on their legislative representative, once again showing the lack of cohesion within the chiropractic community. If an antagonistic chiropractor was a close friend of a committee chairman it normally would mean the death of the bill.

One noon, while having lunch with the executive director of the W.C.A., he was called away to the phone. When he returned to the table, he informed us the bill we had in committee will now be pushed onto the floor for voting. We had been waiting for this for a long time and it was great to hear it would be voted on. Our executive director was asked if the senator said he would put the bill on the floor and he said "no, that was not mentioned". The senator told me he had seen a wonderful John Deere mower with many attachments that he really thought was nice. What this means is, we will deliver one to his home this week, as a gift, and our bill will be released from committee. Welcome to the world of politics. Once the chiropractic profession had increased the dues for its members, it was able to afford the gifts required to pass a bill.

One area the medical profession had developed early in the 20th-century, was the recognition of placing one of their own in the legislative halls. Not only would they have someone on the floor watching the legislative process but also developing relationships with other legislators. This way favors could be exchanged. As president of the Wisconsin Chiropractic Association, I urged the board of directors to establish a program to send chiropractor's to the state legislature. By choosing either, a young graduate with proper credibility or a practicing chiropractor with similar credibility and get all of the chiropractors and their patients to put them in office. The inability of the profession, as a whole, to support one of their own went back to their school affiliation. Some states were able to do this. It should have been done in every state, but the ugly head of school affiliation always surfaced to prevent it being done. There also was an aspect, which came with the investigation. Many rural chiropractors were extremely wary of the larger city chiropractors. This wariness, once again associated with school ties caused many missed opportunities. I was told by a very popular state senator that we could pass almost any bill we wanted if we all got together.

Another aspect covered sponsoring or supporting a candidate campaigning for office. This would seem like a simple process but now we incorporate not only the school allegiance but also the political party differences. So if we had a legislator who always voted for our bills, was a Democrat, the Republican chiropractor would not vote for him. This holds true for Democrat chiropractor's voting for a Republican. It seems ludicrous that professionals, with their profession on the block, would be so juvenile as to consider the legislators party rather than the good of his profession. This can be multiplied over 50 states and you get the same answer. When we did obtain a senator or state representative on the national level they were always admired, but never seemed to take effect on the local level.

Another area of concern was the need for attorneys and executive directors to represent the association. Each state had the same problem. In traveling the 50 states and meeting with State presidents, I found an underlying problem. Many chiropractors, in the 1950's and 1960's were intimidated by attorneys and qualified executive directors. If an attorney, wishing, to represent a state association, said "I believe in chiropractors", the profession would feel he could do no wrong. I saw this frequently, when the attorneys they hired were only interested in their retainers and said, whatever they felt they should say to get the job.

I also proposed to the board of directors that we subsidize a new graduate and send them to law school, with a provision they spend at least five years working for the state association. An opportunity to have one of our own did not take effect. Later one of the practicing chiropractor's did obtain a law degree, on his own, but did not work for the association. This same procedure would hold true in many areas in which the chiropractic profession could benefit.

CHAPTER VII

Medicare-Medicaid Insurance

In the years prior to the 1960's, insurance was not a part of chiropractic practice. In 1953 office calls varied from $1 to a dollar and half. The chiropractic profession was basically unaware of any insurance policies covering health care so it wasn't until the national organizations petition congress to include chiropractic in the new Medicare-Medicaid program. (As the subject was covered to some degree, in a previous chapter,) the medical profession was totally against the inclusion of chiropractic in the program. In discussing this with members of the medical profession, they agreed the problem was bringing chiropractic into credibility with the medical profession in health care matters. It was of no interest to the hierarchy of the AMA if chiropractic was beneficial as a health-care system. The hearings that were held by Congress, were primarily attended by the American Chiropractic Association. There were many individuals in the I.C.A. against insurance programs that would require chiropractor's to follow in medical diagnosis and evaluations. The Congress was very much aware of this division within the chiropractic profession and it was only through grass-roots participation, through-out the United States that was sufficient to have Congress consider the inclusion of chiropractic. Setting up of the rules and regulations, was of course the most difficult part and Congress relied upon the medical profession to provide restrictions and benefits.

Medical testimony had for years been documented indicating there was no such thing as a vertebral subluxation. Once again, it is interesting to note the chiropractic college and medical colleges teach the same subjects, concerning the basic sciences.

First and second year students learn in the field of osteology the segments that are capable of being displaced. The clinical definition of a subluxation means it is less then a luxation or displacement. A dislocation is an advanced stage of a subluxation. In the hearings the chiropractor's, who had a voice representing the profession, apparently were unable to stand up against the medical restrictions and demand equal representation or they felt like Lazarus who could accept only the crumbs offered. Unfortunately, the latter was true and they accepted what ever seemed to be offered.

The most embarrassing requirement was in the field of x-ray when the medical profession convinced Congress that if a subluxation existed it must be confirmed by a medical doctor. The profession that testified under oath that a subluxation does not exist is now asking Congress to allow them to determine whether or not a subluxation exists in a chiropractic X-ray. The X-ray is a primary part of the chiropractic practice because the chiropractor needs this information, based on their schooling, to make a proper chiropractic diagnosis and to determine treatment protocols.

The American Chiropractic Association and International Chiropractors Association should have protested vehemently against this procedure. They did not. I am not sure of the time element but I do feel it was more than five years that every chiropractor taking an X-ray of all Medicare or Medicaid patients had to send that X-ray to a medical doctor to have them confirm whether or not the patient could receive chiropractic care. It was ludicrous. Some medical doctors, the majority of whom never had any X-ray training in medical school were denying chiropractic treatments, losing X-rays or simply not returning them. Still the average chiropractor, happy for the crumbs they had received, felt they had arrived. Whether or not the medical profession, behind-the-scenes, had anything to do with establishing the fee schedule, we will never know. In my discussions with both state and federal politicians, it was confirmed that these decisions are made behind closed doors.

By the 1980's compensation for a Medicare patient was approximately $24.80. In my office, the cost to provide care to one patient was $26.76. When we accepted a Medicare patient, we automatically lost close to $2.00. Medicaid paid slightly over $11.00.

Two paramount controls were added which affected the whole profession. First every Medicare patient had to be X-rayed in order to qualify for Medicare and Medicaid payment. The second part was that Medicare would only pay for 10 visits annually. The patient could attend a medical office 365 days a year for treatment of arthritis and associated symptoms and the medical doctor would be paid for every visit. Though the chiropractic profession was not happy with the restriction felt it was a backhanded compliment by indicating what the medical doctor could not fix in a year, the chiropractor could do in less then ten visits. Many Medicare patients, of lower income could not afford to pay for the X-rays. Chiropractors developed specific office procedures to minimize the number of the X-rays taken, to control the cost and still provide them with enough information for treatment protocols. It was interesting to note when a patient went to the hospital with a neck problem a cervical series (7 views) were taken. The general feeling was the medical profession took films by the pound and the chiropractors took films by the view.

After the federal government passed a Medicare Medicaid law, the states were awakened to the fact that chiropractic, the largest drugless healing profession in the world, was not included in most state contracts. The state legislature determines which insurance companies are allowed to sell insurance in their state. This is regulated by the State Insurance Commissioner. In this instance, the state chiropractic organization began a grass-roots action to be included in all health care policies. For the first time, there was cohesion among the chiropractic profession. Wisconsin was one of the first states to be included in all health care policies sold in the state of Wisconsin. By the 1980's, only 42 states had passed similar legislation. Insurance companies all have on their payroll medical doctors serving as medical directors. As with newspapers and television stations the medical director is to prevent 'snake oil' salesmen from putting them in position to be sued because of an illegal product. The insurance companies immediately set about for loopholes whereby they would not have to cover chiropractic. In testifying before the state senate, I'd listen to testimony from representatives of the Wisconsin State Medical Society; testify that inclusion of chiropractor's into insurance coverage would bankrupt the insurance industry since it would double the cost for every patient. What we had to clarify to the legislative body was how chiropractic would reduce the cost per patient because the patient would not be receiving care in both the medical and chiropractic office and since 85% of patients entering the chiropractic office for treatment leave with reduced symptoms, this will decrease the insurance cost. In addition, the medical procedure requires the insurance company to pay for an office call and in many instances a prescription and/or therapy.

I was part of a committee, formed by the W.C.A to conduct seminars to insurance adjusters and claims officers. The seminars were opened to all health-insurance companies and continued over a four-year period. The purpose of the seminars was to provide information about chiropractic procedures to the attention of those individuals, who authorized payments, for health care, to their insured. The most common question asked was "if the patient is in auto accident and receives evaluation in an ER at the hospital, and then is released without more than first-aid, why is it when they go to a chiropractor one month later they have all types of symptoms which the chiropractor begins to treat. The medical doctor said nothing was wrong".

The answer revolves once again about the lack of education presented to the public. All medical and chiropractic students are aware that immediate trauma causes swelling in the tissues and localized anesthesia. The ER doctor checks for fractures, lacerations, sprains and strains. Finding none the patient is released. After the second week, following an accident, the swelling has reduced and pain, discomfort and limited motion become evident. Not only are these symptoms evident to the chiropractor, but also are visually present on an X-ray.

In order to save the insurance companies money the obvious would be for the ER doctors to refer the patient to a chiropractor before the condition gets worse.

When HMO's became the vogue, chiropractic care was to be included in their plan. Having had firsthand experience with HMO's, I was informed they had found the loophole. The company that covered a large area where I was in practice, fulfilled the letter of the law, that required chiropractic care be available to their insured. They had 225,000 insured customers in our part of the state, so they provided one chiropractor. The letter of the law was followed but not the spirit of the law.

Each state has particular rules and regulations which in turn create their own unique problems. Having taught for over 40 of the state's, and being informed of each state's particular problems, we once again fall back on our national and state organizations who were not providing proper education.

It is interesting to note Wisconsin passed its Workman's compensation law in 1925, allowing full chiropractic care.

Through the 1950's and 1960's, chiropractic students were not made aware of the 'battle' between the professions. There was lack of co-operation between the I.C.A. and A.C.A., the lack of recognition by hospitals, professional sporting teams, industry etc.

I do not know if it would have made a difference in my desire to be a chiropractor but I never would have been made to feel inferior when I naively presented myself in these areas to provide care and treatment. I had been led to understand I was a graduate doctor and as such would receive proper respect and acceptance by the community. Little did I know chiropractors were not always socially acceptable and their children received the same reaction from children of the medical doctor when they were in school. I charge the colleges for not properly preparing their graduates to face the political and social battles that they would be facing in the communities where they established their practice. The battles were far more apparent in the big city areas because of the concentration of doctors and hospitals. The osteopathic hospitals would many times accept chiropractors, as visiting staff. This was evident since the osteopaths were not allowed to practice in the state tax supported hospitals but had to form their own. Therefore, they were sympathetic. I served on the visiting staff of the New Berlin Osteopathic hospital for two years and was able to visit and treat patients. It provided alternative care to the patient and set in my mind the great difference it would make with the inclusion of chiropractic into the medical hospitals.

CHAPTER VIII

Research cooperation
Asthma—Spinal Scoliosis—Allergies

As stated in previous chapters the chiropractic profession began at the beginning of the 20th century, unknown, unlicensed, clinically uneducated and not generally accepted.

Dr. D.D. Palmer had told the early graduates of the Palmer College of Chiropractic to "Go out, heal the sick, and teach". Therefore, by 1906 there were 1000 chiropractors showing up at Palmer College for its annual lyceum. The total number of graduates, by that time, was probably less than a hundred. However, each graduate followed Dr. Palmer's advice and taught everybody, including relatives and friends. There was no research, of any consequence, conducted by the school primarily because everything was so new and there was no grass-roots organization.

I had pointed out that many homes had in their possession two books, one was the Bible and the other was the medical book. The medical book had a variety of homespun treatment procedures for the average household to apply when needed. Some were fairly bazaar such as 'when the patient has consumption, dig a one foot square hole in the yard and have the patient place their face in the hole and breath'.

Since we were basically a rural society, treatment procedures were handed down through the family and were used most often. When the chiropractor recommended adjusting the spinal column to relieve symptoms and correct malfunction, the population readily accepted this principle. As patients would avail themselves to the local chiropractor with a variety of conditions, the treatment protocol was always the same. According to the chiropractors in the first quarter of the century, the philosophy was 'if they are breathing adjust them'. Their basic knowledge of anatomy, neurology, osteology or diagnosis was very lacking. The response to their treatment procedures was phenomenal and by the 1930's many doctors were providing care to over 100 patients per day.

When results fall into the category of 'miracles', the reason why or how did not enter into the equation. When the country went into the flu epidemic of 1917, most patients under chiropractic care never developed the flu. The chiropractor's felt that God had not made any mistakes when he put the body together and if it is functioning normally, the body should be basically immune to disease. D.D. Palmer had even broken the word disease into dis-ease.

The only changes in treatment procedures based on research came about in the field of equipment. The first practitioners practiced in their homes utilizing furniture that was available, such as various types of settees or couches. Individuals designed and built what would be called adjusting tables and by the 1920's companies like Williams Manufacturing developed various types of spring-loaded tables.

One type of research that developed in the 1920's was by Dr. Hugh B. Logan, a graduate of the Universal Chiropractic College. His research, involving many of his colleagues, were concerned about the biomechanics of the spine, and why certain vertebra would rotate out of position, or become subluxated. There undoubtedly were small pockets of research being conducted within the profession but nothing organized under school or state auspices.

The chiropractor in the first half of the 20th-century was concerned primarily with acceptance by the community socially and professionally. Research of any type was left to 'the other guy'. As long as the average chiropractor had great results, they were not interested in knowing why. Some individual chiropractor's did espouse certain procedures they thought wood enhance the treatment of specific cases.

When National College of Chiropractic opened in Lombard Illinois in 1906, a new direction was taken in the profession and some research was begun. Unfortunately, the 'nationalistic' attitude of the colleges did not encourage cooperation.

Dr. Hugh B. Logan's research led to the formation of Logan College of Chiropractic to teach the Logan system of body mechanics, for the reduction of spinal scoliosis and vertebral mal-positions. He founded the first four-year college and did increase the curriculum necessary for a degree.

He established the International Basic Technique Research Institute. Other schools, at the time were still providing only 18 months of education. The utilization of the adjusting table designed by the Williams Manufacturing Company served Dr. Logan's treatment procedures.

Following World War II and the great influx of students into the chiropractic profession with increased educational backgrounds, research did begin. Much research, by doctors in the field with interest towards a particular condition, was disseminated through the clinical journals published for the chiropractic profession. These projects consisted primarily of 'case studies' and recorded results of specific cases. By the 1950's it was surmised there were over 50,000 practicing chiropractor's many of whom subscribe to clinical journals and would be exposed to this information. The schools developed a Post Graduate Program to hold seminars around the country to make some of these studies available. Many of the doctors who had conducted these studies became part of the faculty. The scientific or indexed journals, recognized by the health care professionals in other fields, such as medical doctors, would not accept chiropractic research. The National College was the first college to form a research journal that would be accepted by the scientific community. An interesting example of credibility was when I discussed an article in the indexed Spine magazine, with a medical doctor and he said "it was of no value unless it was in the New England Journal of Medicine".

With the advent of computers in the last half of the 20th-century, it is now possible for doctors anywhere in the world to research articles printed in indexed journals.

Since I was involved with college faculties in the Post Graduate Education Department, I had opportunities to confer with medical research departments. I had published over 30 clinical articles and two in indexed scientific journals and was interested in bringing this information to the medical community. In 1983, after publishing an article on a case study of bronchial asthma, I contacted a bronchial asthma center in Denver Colorado. In talking to the medical director I presented the facts of the case and the results of many cases over the previous 20 years. The medical community had recently published an article indicating a child with asthma could best be treated by removing the child from their home and placing them in an institution. This of course was the article this stimulated my action in calling Colorado. I totally disagreed with that assumption and had clinical proof that chiropractic could not only reduce asthmatic attacks but in some instances removed the condition. The medical director listened to my presentation and then said "in order to have any credibility in your study you must run at least two blind studies". In other words, the work I had done, the clinical research data and the published articles could be thrown into the wastebasket. I was astounded at the response. I was talking to a researcher who may never have been in private practice. I pointed out to him that as a practicing chiropractic physician, located in the same community for over 30 years there was no way I could conduct a blind study, since in my opinion it is immoral. I could not take members of my community, who were suffering from asthma, and in running a blind study, treat half of them for their condition and provide placebo treatment to the other half, still charging them for the visit so they would not be aware they were not really been treated.

Note:

In 2008 the American Medical Association published an article stating that up to 50 percent of the doctors' writing prescriptions were prescribing placebos. Their reasoning was patients always want to receive medication for their problem, and when the doctor does not really know what the problem is; he feels he must prescribe something even though it will be of no value. The AMA stated this is unethical since the doctor is still charging insurance companies for the visit.

I also had the opportunity to discuss the treatment of spinal scoliosis with an orthopedic surgeon, on the board of a Shriner's hospital in Pennsylvania. When I had indicated the number of case studies I had published, he wanted to correlate our findings. Future correspondence indicated he was not allowed to work with a chiropractor.

My experiences in different areas continued to remind me that we were second-class citizens in the field of clinical research. I also had an experience with muscular dystrophy cases as did many of my colleagues. When I conducted seminars around the United States and in other countries, I became privy to much of the individual success chiropractors had with patients. After listening to the muscular dystrophy Labor Day marathon I was taken by the fact, at that time, $423 million had been contributed over the previous 10 years for research into the cause of muscular dystrophy. Interested in bringing the results of chiropractic care into the research program for the benefit of patients, I contacted Jerry Lewis, who as a representative might direct me to the proper contacts. In my opinion, if research is to be done on the cause and effect of a condition, no legal procedure should be ignored. I was told by his manager that Jerry Lewis knew very little about the condition and all the funds were controlled by 18 medical doctors in Boston Mass. The opinion was that I would be wasting my time if I tried to contact them.

Sometimes it is difficult to be exposed to the real world when we naively feel we might be able to help our fellow human with knowledge we have acquired.

It is not all in the medical profession since I was asked to submit a paper to the indexed Journal published by National College of Chiropractic on the subject of spinal scoliosis.

I randomly chose 68 cases from the files and produced a paper showing results of the treatment provided to these cases over a three-year period. Because chiropractic is the only treatment procedure that consistently and predictably reduces spinal scoliosis, the results of my copulation was that, 'we had response in 100% of the cases'. The editorial board of the indexed Journal would not accept the paper because 'it is not possible to have one hundred percent favorable response'. Once again, the lack of information shared between chiropractic colleges brings about professional myopia.

Allergies are another area of concern when it comes to sharing information obtained clinically. When God created a body, he put in some rheostats. Rheostats are familiar to most people's sense that they control the amount of electricity going to light in order to make it lighter or dimmer.

In the body, these rheostats serve to control our bodys's sensitivity to substances.

Example; If one holds a bottle of open ammonia under their nose and takes a breath they immediately will have an allergic reaction notice by burning in the nose and watering of the eyes. This is the body's way of warning you the substance is dangerous. The body responds to various substances by reacting with disturbance in breathing, swelling of eyes, development of a rash, swelling in the throat etc. All of these are set in the body to various degrees in different individuals. All of the reactions are controlled by the nervous system. When anything interferes with the transmission of nerve impulses, it may change the sensitivity of the 'rheostat' making it more sensitive.

Medically the treatment of allergies requires an injection of small amounts of the allergen, to build up immunity. This may take months, years, or a lifetime. Allergies are the easiest to control with chiropractic especially in the area of respiratory. In discussing this response with an allergist, they appeared to be totally incapable of understanding the concept, yet we all studied the same courses.

One experience I had would be typical of an allergy case. A mother brought a seven year-old boy into the office with severe allergies. When I asked what his allergy was, his mother said "dust and airborne pollen". She further stated the doctor wanted her to wash the walls in the child's bedroom everyday. This bothered the mother and gave her reason to call our office. She said the doctor wanted to give the child injections twice weekly and she was never to miss at appointment because it might throw him into an attack requiring hospitalization. I suggested she contact the doctor's office and tell them the child has an infection and that she will call them when the child could come in for his injection. The mother was concerned about the danger of missing the injection. I explained to her that I would be monitoring the case very closely. She agreed and by the time she arrived when he was originally scheduled for his injection, he had been free of any symptoms. I suggested she call the doctor's office again and postponed the next visit, which she did. By the end of the second week, the child was totally without symptoms. I told the mother to come back in two weeks. When she arrived two weeks later, she informed me of her anger. I ask her why and she said "The allergist told me that if he did not get his shots he could end up in a very serious situation. I have missed a total of four weeks and his office has not shown the least concern as to how my son is doing".

Note: Six months later the child still had been symptom free.

I know we do not live in Utopia but considering the health care system today, it would be wonderful if the patient's welfare was the first priority and not the economics. That is why, in my opinion, there will never be a health care system in my lifetime, that will reduce the cost to the patient.

It seems incomprehensible a medical doctor, having spent four years in medical school and a minimum of two years in the residency specialty as an allergist would not be aware of the number of patients who have told them of the results they obtained from chiropractic. I have had discussions with medical doctors and in quoting clinical facts have them say "it is not possible, since there is no published information in the medical journals". The medical doctor is trained to only use acceptable procedures that have been published under medical doctor control. In a recent discussion with an ophthalmologist, I had suggested that increased upper extremity physical exercise causes an increase in the cephalic blood pressure, which is a clinical fact. My assumption was that by increasing this cephalic blood pressure it increases the incidence of 'wet' macular degeneration. He said he could not give an opinion since there have been no published articles on the subject.

My curiosity was aroused by his answer since when one finds repeated results to specific stimuli, it is sufficient to publish an article. The average medical doctor does not publish 'case studies' for the benefit of his profession but leaves that type of thing to someone else. When I suggested he publish a case study based on the information that I had acquired, he indicated he didn't have time. One study has shown that this particular procedure, upper extremity repetitive exercise, does cause an increased incidence of 'wet' macular degeneration. Thousands of individuals with macular degeneration who might I be subjected to strenuous upper extremity exercise, are put in danger of increasing the incidence of 'wet' macular degeneration which leads to decreased vision.

The medical doctor is trained to only accept treatment procedures that have been based on published controlled studies, within the parameters of medical philosophy. A few simple examples will give the reader an understanding of published results in the field of chiropractic that have not been given any consideration by medical researchers.

1. Medical treatment of sciatic nerve irritation (commonly called sciatica) was the injection of alcohol into the nerve, in 1953. In 2008 the only change has been the injection of cortisone.

    a   qualified chiropractor can eliminate the condition in three office calls.

2. The medical treatment for bronchial asthma is the use of bronchial-dilators, and anti-inflammatory inhalers.

    a. Chiropractic care has clinically proved not only reduction in the symptoms, during a severe attack, but of full control of the condition in young individuals without the use of medications. Correction of mis-alignment of the lower cervical and upper thoracic vertebrae releases the irritation of the motor nerves causing the constriction of the alveoli in the lungs, controlling the attack.

3. Medical treatment for low back and hip pain has been physical therapy, injections of cortisone, exercise and surgery.

a. The chiropractic profession has been, not only reducing pain and discomfort for back and hip pain, but has reduced the cause of the condition so as to eliminate the condition completely. This has been going on for over 100 years. Not one medical research program has ever worked with the chiropractic profession to correlate results.

4. The medical profession has been treating headaches with everything from psychiatry to placebos. The frequency of headaches today has mushroomed to what could easily be called an epidemic if it were caused by an organism. I am not talking about brain tumors or cephalic trauma. The universal medical diagnosis is 'stress'.

a. Chiropractic has been reducing and eliminating headaches for over 100 years without the benefit of medications. In 1987 a medical 'headache' clinic in Chicago Illinois reported to the media that their research had proven that the majority of headaches were caused by interference with the nerves coming from the cervical spine. Eureka, the chiropractor's had been saying that for over 80 years but it never made the medical scientific journals. The next 20 years did not produce any follow-up information from that clinic. It could be their findings were outside the medical parameters and therefore dismissed. The state and national chiropractic organizations did not take advantage.

There are not enough free pages in this book to list the hundreds of day-to-day conditions the chiropractic physicians have been treating successfully over the last hundred years but the medical profession is still only providing band-aid treatment.

I have met some medical doctors who have referred patients to chiropractors, for the patients benefit, but I have never been able to sit down with that doctor and discuss the possibility of inter-professional cooperation for the patients benefit.

In the 1970's, I, with members of both the medical and osteopathic profession, formed the Intertribal Medical Missionary Group. Once a month we would fly members of each profession, including nurses, to the Onieda Indian reservation in northern Wisconsin. As professionals, we cooperated in treating the patients based on their need. A medical doctor and I might share a treatment room. The nurse would go to the waiting room, ask if any of the patients had backaches, headaches, leg aches, breathing or stomach problems, and then send them into me. the medical doctor agreed there was nothing he could do for those conditions. He did pap smears and wrote prescription for skin conditions.

The surgeon handled minor surgery problems as they were presented. We worked together within our specialty without animosity to the good of the patient. I had the opportunity to publish an article on the experience, which was ignored by all professions. The Intertribal medical group was disbanded after a couple of years.

In my lecture travels, I did find multi disciplined offices opening up on either coast. In interviewing the chiropractor's in these multi disciplined offices I found it was not as much in sharing their expertise between the doctors as it was in sharing the expense of operating a clinic. (As long as the medical student does not understand chiropractic philosophy, which would have to be presented by their professors, they are incapable of referring on a professional basis. Some medical schools do invite chiropractors to lecture. Once again, the patient is on the short end of the stick.

CHAPTER IX

Public Relations

In the area of public relations, the profession misses the boat in many areas. The loss most noticeable was the 'world posture pageant' founded by Dr. Clair O'Dell from Michigan in the late 1940's.

Logan College of Chiropractic was the first college, to my understanding, to utilize full spine standing X-rays. Medical X-rays have always been classed as sectionals which implied only sections of the body were X-rayed at any one time. The principle behind the full spine X-ray was to visualize the cervical spine and pelvis in one view. The reason for the standing or gravity film was to view the spine in the standing weight position. When the X-rays are taken of the lower or mid back with the patient lying down, the vertebra removed from the weight bearing position tends to de-rotate from their weight bearing position. The medical profession long believed the rotation of vertebra was a compensating factor in posture. The chiropractic profession, aware of the nerve impingement-taking place at the vertebral foramina, was necessary to see the weight bearing position of vertebra.

If a patient had a spine that was in perfect vertical symmetrical position, all the vertebra would be without rotation. Chiropractors had measured the rotation of individual vertebra to determine where the areas of nerve impingement took place. Dr. O'Dell's purpose was to have individual chiropractor's enter patients into a contest to determine which one individual had the 'straightest spine'. The methodology was simple. Each state would determine their representative to compete against other states for the World Posture Queen Crown. The PR potential was significant on local, state and hopefully, national levels. If a state had four districts in the state association, each district would have their own contest utilizing newspapers, radio and television coverage. When it moved to the state level statewide coverage could be obtained. During the times between the 1940's and into the 1970's, pageants of one type and another were frequent. The World Posture Queen pageant utilized appearance, postural attitude and a full spine X-ray. The X-ray was evaluated by a panel of doctors to determine which spine had the minimum number of vertebral rotations. It was a unique contest as the contestants, all female, were interviewed about their experience in chiropractic and were only seen in formal gowns.

Wisconsin participated annually and received television, radio and newspaper coverage.

One of the problems, which developed in the beginning, was that some states had up to three state organizations. In these situations, the state organizations could not agree as to who would sponsor the state contest and in many instances not participate. Once again, it was the failure of the profession by its schools, state and national organizations to instill the need for the good to overshadow the individual.

Some of the cities where the pageant was held were Montreal Canada, Chattanooga, Miami, Atlanta, Los Angeles, St. Louis and San Juan PR. The profession received local newspaper, radio and television coverage in each city but no cooperation from the state association, in which the pageant was held, or promotion by the National Organizations. The pageant was well received by the media and it was the first time chiropractic had been displayed by the media in a favorable light. The pageant was disbanded when the National Organization of Women, (NOW), started demonstrations at other pageants.

Another area that had great PR potential was school examinations for scoliosis. In the 1970's the federal government mandated spinal examinations for grade school children to determine the incidence of scoliosis. The Educational Department did contact the national chiropractic organizations, along with medical orthopedic specialists to determine their participation.

In a previous statement, I pointed out that Logan College of Chiropractic had been founded, primarily on the premises that scoliosis could be reduced under the chiropractic procedures taught at Logan College. None of the other colleges taught the procedure so, the representatives of the National chiropractic association, was not familiar with the Logan procedure and could not agree on how to evaluate scoliosis in the schools. Eventually the medical profession was given the responsibility for the school exams. This fell into disrepute because the medical professionals did not want to leave their offices to go the schools so they would send their nurses, who by the way had absolutely no idea what a scoliosis was. That too became a problem so the doctors' offices recruited mothers to do the examinations with only slight instruction. I do not know how this could have been handled in a worse way, but I do know it was doomed to fail. With the formation of the International Scoliosis Research Center, a chiropractic organization, the schools began calling on chiropractor's to do the physical examinations. Both the A.C.A and I.C.A. were notified by the International Scoliosis Research Center of its existence.

A committee formed of Postgraduate faculty members, who dealt with scoliosis, compiled the chiropractic standards for scoliosis evaluation and treatment. The members of this committee were graduates of different schools but were all nationally and internationally respected teachers and researchers. A copy of the standards were sent to every chiropractic college, both national organizations state associations, and was published in national journals. An ideal opportunity was presented to the profession to move to the fore-front in scoliosis examination and treatment since the medical profession admitted there was nothing they could do other than surgery for scoliosis. Following up in three years after the schools, states, and national groups had been notified, not one group or school could identify the location of the publication. Every student should have been aware of what chiropractic could do for scoliosis and they were not informed. The medical treatment for scoliosis in 1950 included 'wait and see, body braces, and surgery'. In 2008 the procedures are identical and have not changed one bit. In my personal experience of treating scoliosis for over 50 years, I never had a case that did not show some improvement without braces and surgery.

Television opened up an area for chiropractic unprecedented in the previous 80 years. Today, in 2010, chiropractic advertisements are for local doctor's offices. The television industry, along would radio, provides public service announcements (PSA) at no charge. Our national organizations have not provided a nationwide info-mercial on chiropractic. There have been no documentaries on chiropractic success with the treatment of many conditions, no explanation of a chiropractor's education and their specialties. During a six-month period of time, when satellite TV became popular, I had a program called 'Your Healthy Spine' which aired once a week for three minutes. My office was never identified for it was only for patient information about health. Our state organizations also had the opportunity to use P.S.A's but did not take advantage of it. Many actors and actresses, along with producers and directors used chiropractors for their family health but we never see a chiropractor as the main character in a production.

The opportunities passed by do not always keep coming back. I wonder how the national health program would have changed if our national organizations had been the true representatives of the profession and utilized all the opportunities made available.

After retirement, I experienced what could be classed as a cultural shock. Having moved from my home state and relocating in Florida I needed chiropractic care. Recognizing telephone book advertising, for what it is, I attempted to find individuals who had gone to specific chiropractors for a recommendation. I found a few individuals who were not anywhere near comfortable with their chiropractor and very few comfortable with the medical doctor. Since almost everyone is covered by insurance, they had to go to the doctor recommended by the insurance company.

I called three offices on Friday afternoon and received the following announcement "We are closed and if you are in pain please call 911". My training indicated we were doctors 24-7 and not only at our convenience. Somewhere along the line, the schools have neglected to inject the pride associated with being a chiropractic physician. Maybe it's the economic generation who is more concerned about the money. To understand, as a chiropractor, you are able to relieve pain and restore health with the use of your hands. No other profession in the world can attain. It appears the pride and confidence has dwindled, if that was taught in the college, it was lost when they received their license to practice. I do not need to talk about the old days, or what it was like then, but there should be some kind of 'aura' associated with the dedication that should come with the gift of restoring health and relieving pain by the laying on of hands. (Jesus told His disciples to go spread the word, cast out devils and heal the sick by 'laying on of hands').

I have tried to impart to student doctors that there is a gift that comes with their degree. There is no doubt in my mind that individuals who enter the health care fields may well have the gift of healing. Of the thousands of doctors I have instructed, only a small percentage either recognize the gift or become aware of it while practicing their profession. Those individuals are the doctors who love their work, are continually surprised by the response of their patients to the application of their talent. A great surgeon has to be humble when they deal with the inside of the human body and see what God has brought forth. In my experience, I recognize the humility that accompanies the response in the 'laying on of hands'. I was but a young doctor finishing my internship and ready to graduate when this gift was brought to my attention. Many of the students lived in trailer courts, while in college, following World War II. One day there was a knock on our trailer door and a frantic woman's voice called "is anyone home, please answer". In an excited voice, she told me that her six year-old son had drunk from a can of lighter fluid and he had been awake, sitting up for two day's. I inquired as to any medical treatment that might have been applied and she indicated they pumped out his stomach at the hospital, when it happened, and they sent him home. She once again frantically asked if there was anything I could do. Being very young, in the area of experience, other than my internship under a clinic director and an outpatient clinic, I had never treated a patient outside of the clinic. It didn't bother that I was not licensed and it was illegal for me to treat anyone so I agreed to go to her trailer. Obviously, the child was extremely toxic from ingesting the lighter fluid. The hospital physicians did not take this into consideration. I laid the boy on my lap, on his stomach, applied pressure points to areas in his spine and in less the six minutes he closed his eyes and went to sleep. He slept for 18 hours and awoke without residuals. My first, of thousands of experiences, from results of laying on of hands, over the next 50 + years. I was awed by the response and when I discussed this with others, it was apparent many of them had no comprehension of what did happened. Over the years I have met many who recognized this power but unfortunately, in my opinion, the doctors become orientated in the area of economics and in so doing also lose the ability to recognize the gift that has been made available. Because of the chiropractic professions dedication to the application of hands-on approach to adjusting the vertebra of the spine, this gift is manifested on a daily basis. How else could a chiropractor go on a late night house call providing relief to a child suffering an asthma attack, a baby with croup, child with a fever and a woman in labor. To the uninformed reader this may sound far-fetched but trust me, thousands of chiropractors have been doing just this for over a hundred years. This again is why I feel the profession could well have been the leading 'health' care provider. The medical doctor is a 'disease' care provider. Naturally, the surgeons are a necessary specialty, but when you recognize the high percentage of patients realizing immediate relief of their symptoms when visiting a chiropractor compared to the number of patients leaving an internist's office with the same symptoms they had when they entered the doctor's office. Chiropractic works better than many of the chiropractors applying it.

In a book written by James P. Gills, M.D., I quote an excerpt from his book confirming my belief, as I stated before, "the gift of healing is available to all who recognize it and except it." Doctors, because of their calling and daily exposure to individuals who are suffering, become more aware of the gift of healing than the average individual. If they are truly Christian in their heart, they would be aware of the gift of healing available to all.

The following is from Dr. Gill's book:

Faith builds upon faith. As we believe in God and see evidence of His Work, we believe more and have more faith in His power. We also responded with more passion for study in His Word and a greater dependence on the Holy spirit.

Long after his Christian conversion, Tampa cardiologists Dr. Peter Knight witnessed God miraculously heal one of his patients from a disease considered hopeless and terminal. Dr. Knight prayed only for God's will to be done. "I don't ask questions or analyze how", Dr. Knight said.

"I just listen to the Holy Spirit and obey. As I do so, I find my faith to believe for the miracle interesting. Faith builds upon our maturity to stand on His Word and to do what it says". (End of quote from the book)

Once the gift has been recognized the doctor falls into a new category within the healing system. The doctor understands the power of God, the gift of healing, and the application of their talent. Many times over the years, when approached by a patient who responded immediately to treatment, after suffering for a long time, I simply pointed out, with a smile," God does the healing, I just send the bill".

During a patient interview, I tried to inform the patient of all procedures that would follow. I explained how God did not make mistakes when He put the body together and when there is a malfunction, the chiropractor assists the body in recovering. Doctors have long recognized that the patient's attitude has a direct response with their recovery. Confidence in the doctor is paramount. A patients awareness of a positive attitude has an effect on their recovery. If they complain that all is lost without a desire to be better, the chance of correcting the problem is minimized. The doctor may well have faith in their ability and in God's healing power but this must also be transferred to the patient.

The chiropractors that have that phone message to call 911 know nothing of the gift, and their ability to bring relief to the suffering, is questionable.

CHAPTER X

Too late to change back to basics
Truth in philosophy

During the 1970's, the Southeast District of the Wisconsin Chiropractic Association decided to contribute $50,000, in kind, to the American Lung Association. The twofold purpose was to provide chiropractic care in the area of respiratory disease problems, specifically bronchial asthma. The second part was to bring attention of the public to chiropractic's ability to reverse the condition of asthma. The state association was contacted to promote and other states were also encouraged to do the same with the possibility of 50 states offering $50,000 each indicating, to the public, the chiropractic profession's desire to aid the suffering. None of the state's, who were contacted, wanted to participate and the national organizations did not even respond. A large check, 18 in. by 3 ft., was made out to the American Lung Association and arrangements were made to present it at the upcoming American Lung Association fund-raiser. When they were told we would be offering a $50,000 check they enthusiastically set up a time with photographers. When we arrived and were greeted enthusiastically, we positioned ourselves for the picture. The local TV newsreels were there and when we presented the check to the director, we stated "This check for $50,000 is to be used in the South East section of the state of Wisconsin, to cover all expenses, incurred by the American Lung Association, in providing chiropractic care for patients suffering from bronchial asthma".

The director immediately notified the cameras to be turned off and turning to us stated they could not accept the check with those restrictions.

Naturally, it never made the newspapers and try as we may, we could not get them to change their minds.

By the 1970's the course the chiropractic profession had decided to take was too well established to bring about any major change. It is difficult to understand the disjointed internal structure of the profession. I have been privileged to know many of the early leaders in the profession such as: Dr Janse of National College, Drs. Stag and McAndrews of Palmer College, Dr. Vincent Logan of Logan College, Dr. James Parker of Parker College, Dr. Sid Williams of Life College, Dr. Napolitano of New York College, and many others. Each of them a dynamic leader in their own right, but all of them, coming into the profession after the 1920. They were already destined to operate within their own world. As president of the state association, I, and other state presidents did develop a Presidents Association involving the 50 states of the Union. The object was to promote chiropractic's role in the health-care system but unfortunately, at that time, there were still some states where chiropractors were not licensed. The difference in opinions, manifesting themselves in relation to the individual school from which they originated, made the meetings totally ineffectual. Today we do have organizations of college presidents, the Council on Chiropractic Education which grants certification to all the colleges, insurance coverage, Medicare and Medicaid, and Workmen's Compensation coverage for chiropractic care in all 50 states. This is a result more of lay participation into chiropractic care by 'gatekeepers'. Some states were way ahead of others when it came to passing legislation for chiropractors. As an example; as late as the 1970's chiropractors in the State of New York could not X-ray the lower back and pelvis. The state of Mississippi did not recognize chiropractor's as licensed health-care providers. With even this sleight kink in the armor, it was enough so that the leaders in the profession had limited cohesion.

Having lectured for over 40 years on various College Faculties, I had the privilege of meeting many of the clinical leaders in the profession. Most of them had brought the results of their research to the profession through seminars. There were men such as: Drs. Master's, Nimo, Merek, Fuhr, Gonstead and many others. The clinical seminars, unfortunately, opened up the seminars for the promoters. Practice management subjects became up to 60% of the seminar lectures. When clinical subjects, designed to make the chiropractor a more efficient better-trained doctor, are subjected to second place to promoters of equipment and gimmicks, the profession continued on its downward spiral for credibility. With the advent of insurance coverage, the insurance companies began to dictate, not only what type of treatment could be applied, but also frequency and duration of treatment. Doctors by nature, regardless of their profession, are not good at business and consequently are pretty well directed by promoters of new equipment. They also indicate how much more the chiropractor may charge for the service they provide. The state conventions along with the seminars put on by the colleges were easily swayed by the promoters of office management procedures until the younger doctors philosophy was changed from providing health to their patients to how much money each patient would bring into the office.

Chiropractic with its natural treatment procedure did not need all the bells and whistles, which had been proven, in the early years of the 20th-century when all they did was use their hands to relieve suffering. I charge early schools for not making sure their graduates were capable, mentally and physically, to represent the profession. Because all chiropractic colleges are private and did not receive federal funds, it was more important for the schools to have a large number of graduates than to maintain proper standards.

None of the schools prior to 1950 had personal interviews of prospective students by a committee of field doctors to determine their motivation. To this day, only a few colleges do in depth interview with prospective students. That is why the first 50 years of the 20th-century sent the profession on a down hill road to a second-class citizenship.

Is there time to change?

Remembering that following the First World War there were 117 chiropractic colleges and the majority of them were founded for the reason to increase somebody's ego and bank account. There were very few licensing laws in any state so consequently the individual graduates from the schools were released on the public without any control. I spent my early years in a farming community and have always been proud of that time. I do not understand when individuals refer to someone as being a 'farmer' when observing their lack of professionalism. These individuals opened up Chiropractic offices, in back rooms, storefronts, houses and apartments. In the 1950's, I visited chiropractic offices that still had spittoons next to the adjusting table, a coat tree in the waiting room upon which were hanging dressing gowns for women to wear when they received their adjustment. When they finished with their treatment they hung their dressing gown on the coat tree for the next patient. I have been in offices where dogs and cats roam freely through the treatment rooms. I have watched doctors (questionable distinction) smoking during their treatment procedures. The era from 1900 to 1935, created the foundation, (on sand), on which the profession was committed and destined to grow. No firm foundation. Logan College was the first to require a four-year academic schedule. Clinicians were required to wear clinic jackets and to be presentable. Business procedures were instituted into the academic curriculum to get the doctors started in the right direction.

When I graduated, instilled with the pride of my profession, I accepted a position with a chiropractor in La Cross Wisconsin. My expectations were high, I had finished a year-and-a-half of internship and felt qualified to treat patients. Being in-experienced in the quality of doctors in the field, and having been of a generation taught to respect those in authority, I accepted the position with this doctor in hopes of beginning my career. The doctor graduated in 1916 after six months of training in chiropractic and natureopathy. He wore a butcher's apron over a flannel shirt. He had acquired the homespun treatment procedures for his generation. He was as far from my picture of a doctor as one can imagine. I do not blame him for his actions, since his schooling had not prepared him to be a member of a profession. Chiropractors had been accepted in the state of Wisconsin as licensed since 1925 and since this was 1953, I felt he may have acquired more professionalism simply by osmosis. I was wrong. When I came back from lunch one day and found him toweling off and older woman, I questioned what he was doing and he said "We also give baths for 50¢". I left within a week. This was the mentality of that era and when we refer to them as 'farmers' is not in a derogatory way but simply a category of distinction. The man was dedicated, he was very honest and he was concerned, he simply was not professional.

In discussing these points with other clinical lecturer's there was a unanimous agreement that all seminars presenting clinical subjects, particularly at state and college conventions should not include promoters of equipment or management procedures. When the focus is on economics, doctors are drawn to it like a magnet. Many lecturing doctors have seen their class's attended by 30 to 40 doctors when the conference room next to theirs will have 350 attending a lecture on financial rewards by increasing patient load and decreasing the time spent with patients. I heard one management consultant actually say "If you spend more than two minutes with a patient you are losing money".

Is there time to change?

I commend the younger generation graduating today on their professionalism, their academic accomplishments and their motivation. To-day they must have eight years of college plus a minimum of a year's internship. They must pass a three part National Board and the State Board in order to be licensed in any particular state. The generation that graduated prior to 1950 is gone and this generation is building on those who graduated after 1950. Those early doctors obtained what legislation there is, and made inroads in areas that the doctors of today can enjoy. They still are not working together to bring the information to the public of what chiropractic can accomplish. With the American Chiropractic Association and the International Chiropractic Association still having not much more then 30% of the population of chiropractor's to represent, further legislative advancements will be slow to obtain.

There should be a chiropractic department in every hospital with a triage committee, including a qualified chiropractor, to allow chiropractic to minimize hospital stays. Only this generation of chiropractor's can bring this about. As I stated before, with over 1 million new patients per month being accepted into chiropractic offices, the job should be easier if the state and national organizations would combine their efforts for national 'info-mercials' to inform the public of the chiropractic professions ability to reduce health costs and to provide better health care. Recognizing there could be a 38% reduction in hospital occupancy by the use of chiropractic care, it does not set well with hospital administrators and of course becomes a major obstacle. After all, hospitals are a business. You notice the continuing construction around hospitals? Since most of them are classed as nonprofit, they must use their excess funds at the end of the year and what better way than to construct new facilities. I have been on staff of a hospital and have seen how doctors are directed to use certain facilities to increase hospital income.

Medical philosophy emanates from the belief that chemical imbalance brings about disease and the application of medications will alleviate the disease.

Chiropractic philosophy emanates from the belief that the nervous system controls the function of all aspects of the body and therefore if nerves are interfered with, by any means, you may then develop a chemical imbalance. Correcting any interference with the nervous system, specifically through the spine, will allow the body to correct its problem. If medications are used, the combination will be better.

CHAPTER XI

Can Chiropractic be saved?

Conclusion

I recently had the opportunity to observe the Journal's produced by the various chiropractic colleges. As with secular colleges there are those who maintain a slightly higher status. It is obvious the students of today with their eight years of college, minimal one-year internship, three part national boards and state boards, do represent a qualified professional appearance. When looking for a chiropractor, recognize all of them as being qualified, since they have a license. The application of their talent along with their personality determines the quality of the doctor. I am enthusiastic with the quality of these young people that feel they should represent the profession far better than my generation. We recognize the greed that has permeated this generation, in all professions, but with that, set aside, I feel we are going to see more professional offices, with professional caring doctors.

Unfortunately the die has been cast. This younger generation of professionals are going to have to struggle to get the recognition and credibility they deserve since our generation missed the opportunities to move chiropractic into its proper position in the health-care system. As it has been said, 'the children are destined to build upon the sins of their parents'. In this case, our generation dropped the ball and the new generation will be playing catch-up for evermore.

If they can get chiropractic departments in all hospitals, they will be able to gain the recognition they deserve. If the Armed Forces accept chiropractor's in the medical department, commissioning them as officers based on their education, another step towards acceptance will have been made.

I have seen multi-discipline offices containing chiropractors, medical doctors, a physical therapist, and other professionals functioning well together. I feel this may be the best health care system for the patients, allowing them to pick their provider at one location. The biggest stumbling block for this arrangement is the medical profession. I had a medical doctor wishing to practice in my building who was told by the Medical Society of the state of Wisconsin, that she would lose hospital privileges if she were in the same building with a chiropractor. The chiropractor's credibility does not go up by association with the medical physician but it simply provides better care for the patient.

We have chiropractic, radiologists, neurologist, nutritionist, sports specialists, orthopedic specialists, pediatric specialists and family practitioners. Since the medical profession is losing ten percent of family practitioners out of every graduating class, all chiropractors graduate as family physicians so the void can be easily filled.

Conclusion:

Ignored opportunities by chiropractic, lost the chance for a better foothold into the health-care system at the beginning of the 20th-century. We recognize what could have been different if the forces to be had taken advantage of the situation at the time.

What about now? I had mentioned that I would not see a 'patient friendly' health-care system in my lifetime. I had mentioned that the medical profession is not a health care system, but a disease care system. Other than suggestions on diet, exercise and good hygiene, the medical profession simply treats the symptoms of disease until the body heals itself.

The November 2008 issue of Reader's Digest brought up some very interesting points concerning health-care in the United States.

They consider the 'big five' health problems in the country to be coronary heart disease, diabetes, congestive heart failure, asthma, and depression. According to their findings, these conditions account for 75% of the cases treated in doctors' offices. They feel that if there was 1 percent success in the treatment of these cases consistently, it would save $77 billion annually. This is a quote by George Halverson, CEO of Kaiser health systems.

"Considering asthma and diabetes, both of which respond quickly with chiropractic care, the savings might be considered astronomical. Obviously, treatment of the young produces the best results. Chiropractic success is most notable in the young early cases. If a condition is brought under control during early stages of the onset of the condition, the financial savings could be invaluable".

Diabetes is the name of a condition when the cells located in the pancreas, no longer produce insulin to convert sugar into liver glycogen. Medically they try to control the sugar intake and introduce insulin artificially. As I mentioned before, I do not feel God made any mistakes when He put the body together. The nervous system controls the functions of all the cells and chiropractic research has shown mis-alignment of the mid thoracic vertebrae affects the function of the pancreas. In my years in the office, a great number of young diabetic patients had their insulin injections reduced or eliminated under chiropractic care.

If chiropractic and medicine could work together each diabetic patient would receive chiropractic care along with medical care. Since I had previously mentioned how chiropractic can reduce and eliminate asthmatic conditions, the same thing would hold true if both professions worked together with diabetes. If the medical doctor is truly dedicated to the Hippocratic oath the patient's welfare should be the only concern. If the chiropractor treating the case is not capable of correcting the problem, nothing is lost.

Considering the merging of two licensed recognized professions for the treatment of asthmatics and diabetics, a major breakthrough would be made with our health care problem. In 2008, diabetes was considered the fastest growing condition in the United States.

Based on a report from the American Medical Association, approximately 100,000 patients die per year, from medical mistakes primarily known as 'Iatrogenic' disease, (Doctor caused). This statement was recently quoted from the C.E.O. at Mayo Clinic. In my early years I frequently heard medical spokesmen speaking of the number of patients killed under chiropractic care. In my years of lecturing around the world, conducting research for publication and investigating these reports, I was only able to confirm two cases of cervical trauma to a patient by a chiropractor. In both cases, the chiropractor did not evaluate the case properly. I had mentioned, if we consider the approximate 50,000 practicing chiropractors who treat in excess of 10 million patients per month, it justifies why the malpractice insurance premiums for chiropractors, has remained low.

Billions of dollars are wasted on the wrong diagnosis resulting in incorrect medications and in some cases disastrous results. If the medical profession and the chiropractic leaders could combine talents and allow for second opinions, it would be to the patients benefit. When I discussed the work we did with intertribal medicine and how all the doctors worked together, the advantage to the patient was obvious.

There have been many cases, usually taking place in small towns and rural areas, where chiropractors and medical doctors have worked together in a limited way. I know of medical doctors, who would refer musculoskeletal conditions, such as backaches, shoulder and leg problems, to the chiropractor. This was always for the patients benefit. It could have been enlarged at the correlation between chiropractic care in preventing disease with medical treatment procedures. In the early 1900's National College of chiropractic did participate in the Medical College by observing surgeries. Today we have found some medical schools inviting chiropractors to provide medical students with information on chiropractic. It is a foot in the door but no great break through for the patient. The armed services have been petitioned to include chiropractic as part of health care system. In the 40 years, since the first recommendation by the chiropractic profession was made, nothing has been accomplished. If chiropractors were allowed to practice in veteran's hospitals, as well as civilian hospitals, a 36% reduction in hospital stays would be noted. What if the government would institute a program where all practitioners would be required to post the treatment protocol and results of that treatment protocol, into a nationwide computer program for immediate access by all doctors. If this included all the primary care doctors and chiropractors, the information obtained would be monumental. Statistics have shown primary care medical doctors have a 35% success rate at reducing patient symptoms at the first visit. Chiropractic has 84% reduction of patient symptoms at the patient's first visit. As it has been said most often, it doesn't take a rocket scientist to come to a proper conclusion.

I have personal friends who are taking in excess of 12 medications per day. Clinicians will tell you any individual consuming six or more medications per day will cause liver and kidney damage. These are two personal friends, multiply that by millions and you see why our mortality rate is so high. We have the highest infant mortality rate of most civilized countries.

I devoted over 40 years of research into sudden infant Death syndrome (S.I.D.S.). Medically the condition is classed as 'idiopathic', (unknown cause), and yet the chiropractic profession has shown the condition is predictable and correctable. Over 5000 children die per year diagnosed with S.I.D.S and yet there never has been a chiropractic treated baby die of this condition. The cause of SIDS is the obstetrical practice of head rotation during the birth process. This has been confirmed clinically by medical and chiropractic researchers. The chiropractic national associations have not taken the opportunity to bring this information to the public. Discussions with the medical community have been met by closed doors.

The emergency rooms in the local hospitals are over burdened and under staffed. Young uninsured families use the ER as their doctor. Many communities have established small local walk-in clinics called 'docs in a box'. They are an answer to the overcrowding in the ER but allowing chiropractor's in the ER to provide care for musculoskeletal conditions could greatly improve over crowding. With less medical school graduates going into primary care, each year the system has noted over a 10% drop in primary care physicians from 10 years ago. Some legislators are suggesting loan forgiveness in order to entice medical doctors to go into primary practice. It would be nice if they would open their horizons to include the chiropractic students of which over 80 percent go into primary care.

In December 2008 a newspaper in Ocala Florida, the Star Banner, carried an article concerning the family care physicians in Florida. The organization of family care physicians noted a 29% decrease in their income from Medicare and Medicaid over the last three years. Each of the last three years has shown a reduction in the amount of money paid to the doctor for Medicare and Medicaid patients. There are 111,000 primary family care physicians in Florida and they have taken into consideration a policy to refuse to accept any Medicare and Medicaid patients in the coming year. I can relate to this. While in practice, I accepted Medicare patients and found that it cost, at that time, $25.16 to treat one patient that was on Medicare. Medicare paid me $21.50 so in effect; I lost money with each patient. Medicaid paid $11.50 for each patient. This was over 30 years ago when office calls were less than $30 per visit. With today's operating expenses in any office it is understandable why 111,000 primary physicians would refuse to except Medicare and Medicaid patients.

The health-care system will be continually covered with Band-Aids to try to stop the hemorrhaging. It will not help. It may take a government mandate to require all licensed health-care professionals' access to all tax supported hospitals and research facilities.

There is no 'imprimatur' for this book, because it enters into an area that holds hundreds of years of discrimination. As stated earlier, if a 'Triage' were set up in every hospital for evaluation by both professions, our health care system would improve immediately.

In the early years of the 20th-century, many chiropractors were being arrested for practicing medicine without a license. Palmer College of

Chiropractic formed a club called the 30-60-90 club. If you were arrested for practicing without a license and sentenced to 30 days, you could be a member of that club, etc.

Remember, the majority of chiropractor's were located in the midwest, particularly Iowa, Wisconsin, Illinois, Minnesota and Missouri. There was no licensing prior to the licensing law that was passed in Wisconsin until 1925. The chiropractor's of that day felt it was a badge of honor to be arrested for helping the sick to be relieved of their problem.

It became so common by the 1930's that one event that took place in Rice Lake Wisconsin, according to observers, spread through-out the profession. Dr. I. N. Toftness, who had a successful practice in Rice Lake, was well known and respected. The county medical society filed a complaint that he was practicing medicine without license and he was brought before the local judge. The judge asked him what day of the week his office was closed and Dr. Toftness responded, 'Thursday'. The judge stated he would confine him to jail each Thursday for the next month and that he could bring his adjusting table to the jail to provide care for his patients. When word got around the patients lined up at the jail to receive their care.

If the pharmaceutical companies could convince the chiropractic profession to write prescriptions there would be a full endorsement by the pharmaceutical community for chiropractic. Unfortunately, for those companies, the chiropractic profession, at this time, has no interest in writing prescriptions.

On December 8, 2008, ABC news commented on two health issues. One stated that 32% of the population has fore-gone traditional medicine and is using alternative care, such as chiropractic, for their health care. The second statement indicated over 34% are moving into vitamins and health foods and using fewer prescription medications. In December 2008, ABC reported there were 11,000,000 back surgeries in 2008, with less than a 1% permanent relief noted by the patients. At approximately $50,000 per surgery, how much might have been saved with a 'triage' department. Maybe it is not too late to change!

The opinions I have presented in this book are derived from my experiences as a family practitioner, specialist in scoliosis correction and postgraduate faculty member, accumulating over 56 years in the profession. I do not intend to change individual opinions about the profession of chiropractic but to inform those interested in the profession, as to what shaped chiropractic's destiny.

Summary

1895 A new procedure for treating health problems was initiated by David D. Palmer a magnetic healer in Devonport Iowa.

1896 the new procedure was named Chiropractic from the Greek word 'Chiro' meaning by hand and 'practic' for the word practice.

1897 B.J. Palmer, son of D.D. Palmer, convinced his father to begin the school for the teaching of chiropractic.

1902 Workers' compensation law is established. Neither B. J. nor his father recognized the need for chiropractic to be included, in this legislation, primarily because licensing laws had not been established and because the mentality of the day was to 'take care of yourself'.

1906 D.D. and B.J. Palmer form the Universal Chiropractic Association. Note: The author has been unable to determine the motivation for the formation of the Universal Chiropractic Association other than the possibility of maintaining control over the profession's growth.

1908 Two more colleges were formed. National College in Lombard Il was one of them.

1909 B.J. Palmer developed the Meric theory. Since nothing had been written about this new technique, chiropractic, B.J., being a promoter recognized the need to have what the college teaches, recorded. The Meric system established a correlation between the nerves emanating from the spine to their point of innervations. This information, put into book form in later years became the 'Bible' for many practicing chiropractors. If the patient was a man with stomach ulcers, the Meric theory indicated the patient should be adjusted in the area of the fifth to seventh thoracic vertebrae. If the patient had lung problems, adjustment of the vertebra from the fifth cervical through the third thoracic, would be indicated. The theory, substantiated by neurology in later years, continued in use through the 1960's. In reality, it isn't completely accepted by the profession and is not practiced by the newest generation of chiropractor's. This theory, some feel was divinely inspired, for it simplified cause and effect. Recognizing, as an example, bronchial asthma manifest itself by the patient being unable to exhale the air that is in their lungs. The controlling factor is a muscle located at the entrance to the alveoli that goes into constriction preventing air from leaving the lungs and forcing the patient to constrict their chest muscles to expel the air, causing a rasping sound. The control for this muscle is located in the area of the first and second thoracic vertebrae and if pressure is applied at that point during an attack, the muscles relax and the breathing becomes normal. Chiropractors treating asthma cases became very familiar with the quick response to this treatment.

1919 Three more chiropractic schools were opened. At this time, if it would have been brought to the attention of B.J. Palmer, considered the leader in the profession, to correlate the educational criteria, the health-care field would be in a different place today.

1922 B.J. established a radio station in Davenport Iowa. Again, we find the possibility for instruction of the population as to the benefits of chiropractic. The direction of the information was towards the population, which increased the acceptance by the people. It is unfair for us to try to determine what was in their mind that the time, but hindsight, and 80 years later we can see what opportunities were missed. Ronald Reagan obtained his first job as a radio announcer on that station.

1924 B. J Palmer develops the Neurocolometer. This instrument measures the heat hrough two prongs, on either side of the vertebral column, indicating possible nerve flow disruption. When I wrote the first volume on the history of chiropractic in Wisconsin, I interviewed doctors who had graduated in the 1920's. The majority pointed out that they were required to purchase this instrument, before they graduated, and not too share it with anyone who was not a Palmer graduate. This attitude manifested itself in all schools. Each school would try to develop a new procedure which they could keep to themselves to enhance their school.

1926 B. J. Palmer established the International Chiropractic Association. Looking back over 80 years, B.J. Palmer, the strongest leader in the profession, could have required every college and all students to belong to the association to build a powerhouse. I recognize I am being naive.

1930 B.J. Palmer develops the 'Hole In One' theory. This procedure dealt with specific adjusting of the first cervical vertebra, which implied it affected the rest of the body. The theory was not shared with any other college.

1930 The National chiropractic association was formed.

1941 Accreditation was granted to the chiropractic profession by the United States government.

1944 The United States government began to fund research. Because there were remnants of the Universal Chiropractic Association, International Chiropractic Association and the National Chiropractic Association, there was no universal approach to obtain funds, for research in chiropractic. This was one of the greatest errors committed by the profession's early leaders. The profession was spending all its time treating people in individual offices without ever trying to provide a unified front to prove what they were doing was correct and at the same time enhance their place in the healing arts.

1947 History was able to reach a milestone when one particular chiropractor became the most jailed chiropractor in the United States. Though it means nothing by itself, it indicates the profession was considering being jailed a joke, rather than the dangerous precedent it was establishing.

1961 saw the establishment of the Medical Congress on Quackery. Its prime, and only mission, was to eliminate chiropractic as a health-care provider. The leaders of the chiropractic profession ignored the formation of the Congress and went about their daily practice, apparently feeling if they ignored it, it may ago way.

1963 The A.M.A. declares war on chiropractic. The chiropractic profession turns its back and goes about its business. By this time there are over 50,000 practicing chiropractors taking care of millions of patients. The leaders in the chiropractic profession probably felt they were well established. Most states had licensing laws protecting them from being arrested but they were unaware their position on the health provider latter was being lowered a step at a time.

1960's saw the formation of Medicare and Medicaid. This was discussed earlier in the book but it suffices to say the profession being so fractured without any unified front, would allow the medical profession to dictate whether or not the chiropractors were to be accepted into Medicare and Medicaid programs. The medical doctors testified before Congress that there was no such thing as a subluxation (displaced vertebra).

Congress agreed to have chiropractor's included in Medicare and Medicaid, to adjust mal-positioned vertebra. The medical representatives convinced Congress that first, all chiropractic patients must be X-rayed, at their own expense and that the X-rays must be sent to a medical doctor to determine if a subluxation exist. Then they convinced Congress that they could only allow Medicare patients ten visits per year to a chiropractor. A patient may visit a medical doctor 365 days a year and have each visit paid for by Medicare. Unaware of what restrictions were being placed on the profession, the leaders in the chiropractic profession took this to mean that chiropractors were so good they could correct a problem in ten visits when it would take a medical doctor one year to correct the problem. The chiropractor's attitude seemed to be 'just give us something'.

1975 Chiropractic Research began to be published in clinical magazines. There were no scientific journals (medical) that would accept a chiropractic article. The scientific community does not accept a clinical article as scientific proof. Their criteria had been established by the pharmaceutical companies, who provided not only the funding but also most of the research for any scientific article. This again was not available to the chiropractic profession since they were fractured as to their unified presentation of need for scientific research.

1976 Dr. Chester Wilk, an Illinois chiropractor filed a Federal Discrimination suit, in federal court, against the American Medical Association for discrimination. The court ruled in favor of Dr Wilk.

1988 merger talks of the ICA and ACA failed. It is hard to understand how after 80+ years of dis-unification that the leaders of the chiropractic profession would be continually ego centered and continued to sacrifice their profession. When I was president of the state association attending a national meeting of presidents I was appalled by the individuals manifesting their superiority over other states without any indication for unification.

After 57 years in the practice of chiropractic I can think of no other way that I would like to have spent my life. I have had many conversations with members of other professions particularly with members of the medical profession. I have had close relations with surgeons, pediatricians and general practitioners. The majority of those individuals indicated to me that they would not encourage their children to follow them in the medical profession. Primarily this has to do with the bureaucracy, paper filing, increased harassment by government officials and the dependence of the medical profession upon drug companies to tell them how to run their practice and treat their patients. The joy I found in working with people over the years came from the personal attention that I was able to provide the individuals. My 47 years in private practice, in the same community, allowed me to appreciate small town health care. I made house calls on the average of once a day. Many of these house calls were in the middle of the night because; as the medical profession changed they were making fewer house calls. I remember one young medical doctor telling me he was going to triple his fees for house calls to discourage people from calling him. He surprised me since I was still young enough to feel that we were dedicated doctors 24-7. I will probably repeat myself many times but one of the problems with chiropractic and is that it is so simple. I would go on a house call with nothing other than my hands and would be able to relieve pain, restore breathing to an asthmatic, reduce the fever in an infant, and do a variety of other symptom reductions. The satisfaction gleamed from that made the profession worthwhile. There are hundreds of cases I could talk about. The response I received from patients astounded me in the early years and I recognize the medical doctor's giving someone a medication and then leaves asking them to check again to see if there had been any change. The response I received was always immediate. When we begin dealing with cause and effect and allow symptoms to direct us where the cause may be located, treatment of the problem becomes much simpler. I know that you feel this has always been the way doctors treat conditions but if that were true, I would not be writing this book. The medical doctor (internist) is trained to look for a chemical imbalance cause, and treat from that standpoint. The medications either stimulates or inhibits body function. For example, if you take a pain pill, it nullifies the transmission of pain impulses to the brain. If you take insulin, it stimulates the body to convert sugars to liverglycogen.

In the nineteen forties and nineteen fifties, many states did not have licensing laws for chiropractors. This was the fault of not only the state organizations but of the National organizations, American chiropractic association, and the International chiropractic association. There was some activity by both the state and national organizations but it ended in divisive action by the opposing individuals concerned with philosophy. The philosophical divisions in chiropractic had to do with specific adjusting of the vertebra and those doctors who wish to use various types of therapeutic equipment. Looking from the outside, it seems like a silly reason to cause a fight. Because there was no direct leadership from the national organizations, the individual squabbling in the state's continued. The last state to license chiropractors was the state of Mississippi. When Mississippi granted a license to chiropractors they included a grandfather clause to anyone who had been practicing some type of health procedure. This never should have been allowed. Their were individuals who were simply massage therapists and were given a chiropractic license, even though they had never attended one day of school. I feel the state and national organizations should have worked together to prevent this type of miscarriage of justice to the patient.

History books have indicated that during the Civil War, more soldiers died from infections and surgeries than on the battlefield. It was stated a good surgeon could amputate a leg in ten minutes. Service personnel returning from World War II had seen a great improvement in medical procedures since the Civil War and many were anxious to get into the chiropractic profession. The inability of the national organizations and the schools to prepare for this influx became obvious. They should have been assured of government support for the applicants to chiropractic college. Years later, the Consul on chiropractic education was formed to accredit colleges. By this time, too many schools had graduated individuals who were not truly qualified in the field of chiropractic.

When doctor D.D. Palmer testified before the legislative house in Iowa concerning chiropractic, he made the statement that he could teach a person to adjust the spine in 30 days. Since the practice of chiropractic had to do with the adjusting of the individual vertebral segments, teaching the procedure was not that difficult. We understand there is much more to treating the sick and simply adjusting the vertebra, but his point was that it was not that complicated. It would equate to be able to teach a medical doctor to write a prescription in 30 days. There is also more to the practice of medicine than writing prescriptions. One of the big complaints voiced by the medical profession, 100 years ago and still today, is that chiropractic delays proper medical care and can cause injury. First of all a chiropractor cannot adjust the vertebra that is in the proper position and secondly they are not preventing proper medical treatment, they are correcting the cause of the problem.

I had mentioned in chapter two about doctor Morikubo of La Cross Wisconsin, who was accused of practicing medicine without a license. There were no licensing laws in Wisconsin at that time and because of the media discussing the possibility of war with the United States against Japan, the medical profession determined it was a good time to go after this Japanese chiropractor. I practiced in La Cross Wisconsin and interviewed doctors who had been in the community for many years. They informed me that members of the medical profession had told them they were determined not to let any other health practitioner treat the sick. They took advantage of the media's interest in the Japanese to accuse this individual practicing medicine. The state legislature determines the scope of practice of anyone in the health field. The scope of practice for the medical doctor is open. In specialty areas such as optometrists, massage therapist, and dentists, they are limited to the specific area in which they work. Only the chiropractor, osteopath, and medical doctor are allowed to treat the sick from head to foot.

When the medical profession accused Dr. Morikubo of diagnosing, it implied that any parent who diagnoses their child of having a head cold fever or possible infection is practicing medicine without a license. The jury in the trial recognized immediately what the medical profession was doing and found the doctor not guilty. As I had mentioned, this was a red flag, a warning that should have been evident to the leaders of Palmer college and of National college that there was a battle that was about to take place to discredit the chiropractic profession.

I recognize that because of school policies, some students were accepted with less than an eighth grade education and it would take years for the profession to recognize the need for more education. Those who were practicing with limited education would fight to keep there license. Education develops maturity and thought in action. Even though the practice of chiropractic did not require advanced academic education, it did require mental maturity.

In later years, when I testified before the Wisconsin state senate committee on health, it was brought to my attention the lack of education of many of the chiropractors practicing in Wisconsin. The first doctor I went into association with was a 1916 graduate of a naturopathic school with six months of education. He produced results with patients because of the simplicity of chiropractic philosophy. His methods of practice fell far below what we would consider to be professional. Many times it appeared that patients came by the busload since he was always busy. This did cause confusion in the medical profession because they knew his background and could not understand how he could produce such results.

Today, they should well understand that the chiropractor and a medical doctor have the same basic training in their graduate studies. Chiropractors do not study surgery or pharmacology to any extent. The medical profession does not spend much study time on musculoskeletal conditions.

To-date, the profession is licensed in all fifty states, accepted in insurance plans, being utilized in professional sports, and mentioned in TV sitcoms. Efforts are continually being made to get them in hospitals. Regardless of the populous acceptance, all of these changes still regulate them to the same category as 'physical therapists'.

As they say in jurisprudence, 'Res Ipsa Loquitor'. The situation speaks for itself.

The End